How to Find A Dominant

Common Sense Tips for Submissives Interacting On and Offline

by

Jude Samson

Moons Grove Press
British Columbia, Canada

How to Find A Dominant:
Common Sense Tips for Submissives Interacting On and Offline

Copyright ©2019 by Jude Samson
ISBN-13 978-1-77143-395-2
First Edition

Library and Archives Canada Cataloguing in Publication
Title: How to find a dominant :
common sense tips for submissives interacting on and offline / by Jude Samson.
Names: Samson, Jude, 1979- author.
Identifiers: Canadiana (print) 20190130962 | Canadiana (ebook) 20190130997 |
ISBN 9781771433952 (softcover) | ISBN 9781771433969 (PDF)
Subjects: LCSH: Sexual dominance and submission.
Classification: LCC HQ79 .S26 2019 | DDC 306.77/5—dc23

Cover artwork credit: Woman in handcuffs, Man in handcuffs, slaves
© KlausHausmann | Pixabay.com

The BDSM Emblem image is copyright 1995, 1997 by Quagmyr@aol.com who maintains the copyright in order to protect the symbol, and is used herein by permission. The explanatory text is copyright 1995-2013 by Quagmyr@aol.com, and is used herein by permission.

The pony-play image is copyright Tigger, and is used herein by permission.

All other images contained herein are either copyright Jude Samson or are in the Public Domain, and the latter are used without malice.

Disclaimer: Extreme care has been taken by the author to ensure that all information presented in this book is accurate and up to date at the time of publishing. Neither the author nor the publisher can be held responsible for any errors or omissions. Additionally, neither is any liability assumed for damages resulting from the use of the information contained herein.

Moons Grove Press is an imprint
of CCB Publishing: www.ccbpublishing.com

Moons Grove Press
British Columbia, Canada
www.moonsgrovepress.com

Dedication

First and most importantly, I'd like to give a resounding thank you to my friend and proofreader LucsCarolinaJoy who worked tirelessly to make this book legible. She embraced my voice, understood the tone, and did an amazing job to make sure everything sounds just right.

I'd also like to thank my friend Tigger for allowing me the use of his pony image.

I would also like to thank Quagmyr for allowing me the use of the BDSM Emblem image and definition.

This book is dedicated to everyone who helped me over the years on my own personal journey of the lifestyle.

It is also dedicated to my dear friends, you all know who you are, who have taken me under their wings, invited me into their lives and families, and through their example have shown me what it means to be a dominant and a good person. Additionally, they have given me their kindest support in this endeavor whether in purchases, auction-winnings, or feedback to make it even better than ever.

Initially, this book was also dedicated to all the "trolls" who seem to fill the inboxes of female dominants across the globe. In fact, they prompted this venture. But upon its release, I have received some wonderful responses from genuine men who found this information helpful in setting them in the right direction. So this is now also dedicated to those who truly seek to better themselves as life is a constant journey of self-exploration and I give you a great deal of credit for your efforts.

About Sir Jude

In my 20+ years in the lifestyle, I have grown from an awkward beginner into an active dominant in my local community. As I was Assigned Female At Birth (AFAB) I didn't know what transgender was and so I was a lesbian dominant and often just said that I 'male-identified' and, as such, preferred all terms, pronouns, and references to be masculine. The community around me was amazingly accepting and freely used any gender or terms I (or anyone else) wanted and, in fact, it was at a munch where someone first told me the word I was seeking was "dysphoria." Because of the community (with a few exceptions) I finally felt ready to take the step to transition from female to male (FtM).

As I developed an understanding of the D/s lifestyle I discovered I'm far more interested in the strict structure of the Master/slave relationship. I have learned a great deal over the years about BDSM, about scenes, the tools of the trade, and various aspects of play and the dynamic between dominant and submissive. I feel there will never be a point in my life when I will stop (nor want to stop) learning about myself, my kink, and the world around me.

I find I have a unique ability to step back from situations to observe the delicate interactions that take place in the lifestyle and have used those observations to contribute to a lot of forum topics, articles for my personal website, in developing a household manual, and now in writing this book.

I feel it's vitally important to share the information that I've gained with the community at large. There is no reason or point to hoarding information, advice, or guidance within the community and I actively engage in teaching whatever I've learned.

Lastly, while this is the first edition of *How to Find a Dominant* the bulk of the content is originally from *How to Find a FemDom* that I wrote in 2012 (1st edition) and 2013 (2nd edition). Needless to say, a lot has changed in the over six years since I first started writing this in the overall BDSM culture, Internet sites, and apps. Additionally, the information contained really fits with any gender of dominant or submissive so I reworked it to be more gender-inclusive/non-gender specific.

Contents

SECTION THREE:
OFFLINE/REAL LIFE COMMUNITY

SECTION FOUR:
MEETING A SPECIFIC DOMINANT

SECTION FIVE:
IN-HOME SERVICE

Introduction & Purpose

There is no magical sequence of events that
will be 100% guaranteed to get you that perfect dominant.

Good, now that we've gotten that squared away, we can talk a little about the real purpose here and how it's meant to help you, the prospective submissive.

I've seen more and more submissives lament, "Why is it so hard to find a dominant?" This is often posted in various BDSM related groups/forums and it's a lament echoed by submissives and slaves of all genders. However, on the opposite side of things dominants also complain about the piss-poor quality of messages they receive and contacts they have with "so-called" submissives.

What does this all boil down to? It's a numbers game mixed with a bit of a society that is increasingly more concerned with cutting corners, saving time, and putting in half-efforts, but expecting maximum results. Let's break it all down. I'm going to discuss not only all the things that are done wrong but also important things to watch out for in order to protect yourself (and your privacy), how to avoid scams, and how to do things right.

The numbers game: Surprise, surprise! The "common" mixes are male submissives seeking just women (or a female-led couple), female submissives seeking men only (or male-led couples), men seeking men, and then women seeking women with bi/pansexual submissives seeking a dominant of any gender - and that's just counting those who are genuinely seeking to submit in real life. Also, throw in all the HNGs (Horny Net Geeks) and Wannabes who want a quick online jerk-off that seem to outnumber the genuine seekers. Between the fakes and the "real" submissives, you're talking about massive submissive overload. In fact, it's because most of the fake ones filling up our inboxes that the ones who are truly sincere in their desire to submit get lost or accidentally discarded. A submissive doesn't just have to woo a dominant using only the power of their words in that first email exchange, they also have to compete with the countless other emails coming in that are, simply put, junk.

As a submissive gets more discouraged by this lack of instant gratification, they tend to resort to mass-emailing by sending a cut-and-paste form letter to every single person who has "dominant" in their profile. Even, on occasion, sending them to submissives or those of the gender they are not interested in just because the word dominant is somewhere near the top of the profile and that's as far as the lazy submissive has read.

Regardless of whether it's a matter of being disheartened or of being an HNG this is *not* the path to take. I'll talk about this in further detail later, but remember, the submissive needs to stand out, not blend in with the "losers" to even get a response, much less eventually attain a successful D/s relationship.

Unfortunately, the ones who need to read this... won't

I hear this frequently when I've posted tips and other advice in forums. The actual answer is – if they need it but **won't** read this (or any other research) then they're probably not the ideal submissive right from the start. If they are sincere about their submission and might be just a little misguided, then a gentle leading to this book or other online resources will result in that submissive doing their homework. **They** are the one we will be more apt to work with and take into our lives and it is **them** that this book focuses on guiding.

I have seen submissives who were new to online sites read posts along these lines and then watched their profiles and manners drastically change to reflect this new insight. It does work... if the submissive is genuine and willing. If they are not... then they can simply go into the dismissed pile like the rest of them.

Submission is work... get used to it

There may be times your entire reward will be your dominant's hand patting your head or hearing, "Good boy/girl/sub/slave." There are times when your dominant may do something that you truly love and enjoy as their way of showing how much they appreciate what you do for them. These little moments bring pleasure, a heated glow, a deep stirring of happiness. It's when you expect or demand reciprocation in some form that this becomes more of an arrangement with a Pro-Domme or when you may want to seek out specific fetishists rather than promote yourself as looking for someone to serve. Don't get me wrong, the submissive has needs and desires too and those need to be taken into account and discussed over time with equal importance, but remember, a submissive is ultimately there to be of service. The crux of a D/s dynamic, however, is to submit oneself to the will of another. It's ensuring you've picked the right dominant who has interests and kinks that are aligned with your own that provides the fulfillment of all the little things that get your blood pumping. This is not necessarily a dynamic of equality in the more common sense but rather a willful exchange of power to purposefully create an inequality (or, at least the overall sense of inequality). There are just varying degrees to how "unequal" your dynamic is based on what you're both seeking but in the end, it is a life of strength, not weakness.

True strength lies in <u>submission</u> *which permits one to dedicate his life, through devotion, to something beyond himself. (Henry Miller)*

What This Book Is NOT:

I don't want anyone reading this to assume that by buying this book and going through it, no matter how many suggestions you may follow, that you are guaranteed to find your perfect dominant. Even if you follow this book to the letter there is no way to promise you'll find your dominant by the time you reach the end, or even for a long while after – there's just simply no way to guarantee something like this.

This is a general guide and, as such, results will vary. As each person is unique, what one person can make seem endearing or funny another could just as easily make it seem soiled or creepy. I cannot, and will not, give you a play-by-play guide because it would be impossible. To garner the most from this book you should take a close, introspective look at yourself and during that process try to discover how the external world views you, and then utilize the guides and tips herein to increase your odds of success. Besides, not only will self-reflection help you in your daily life as a human, it will be a skill that will guide you in finding a dominant partner and in maintaining a healthy relationship.

Realize that these are suggestions, tips, and warnings that have been compiled from firsthand accounts relayed by dominants as well as some of their wants, suggestions, and desires as to how a would-be submissive should present themselves or behave. Many submissives have offered tales of struggle in the seemingly daunting search for a dominant. I have tried to objectively provide the best advice available, but remember that ultimately you are the master of your own fate… at least until you surrender it.

One of the most recurring things you will see throughout this book is "if you do a search for…" and I make that statement repeatedly because it seems that people refuse to access the knowledge that is at our fingertips. I have often written/emailed/texted something that referenced a place, person, or general subject that the other person didn't understand. Instead of being lazy and asking "who is that" or "what's that mean" just take a split second to search online to find out for yourself. Use the knowledge at hand rather than taking the "I don't know," or "who is…" approach.

While I do include a brief chapter about serving a dominant and some general expectations and warnings when you reach that goal, this is not a training manual that will give explicit details on how to serve. Why? Because every single dominant is different and there are so many varying degrees of D/s that each and every dominant will want you to act, react, and behave in different ways to their personal taste. Although I am not focusing on this aspect of service training, there are resources provided in the final chapter to help you acquire skills that would be of service to a dominant. While some of the topics or skills may seem mundane or be things that some people "should just know" there are fewer and fewer people who hone and utilize these skills and the art of service is quickly vanishing.

My point, at its simplest, is to give you a general idea of things to avoid, areas to improve, what you should be doing, and how you should be doing it in order to have a _**greater chance of success**_.

What makes finding the dominant you want to serve so difficult, is that you are looking for someone who has the same desires you have, but from the opposite side of the slash in a sea churned up and filled with rubbish and now requires far more attention to detail and careful navigation to make that journey.

FOR EXAMPLE:

If you have a huge foot fetish where you like to suck, rub, and have a person's foot anywhere and everywhere all over your body, you are narrowing your search to someone who wants all of those things done to them. If you crave the crack of a single-tail, then you are narrowing the search to not only someone who likes them too, but someone with the skill to wield one as well.

It's not necessarily that the ratio of dominants to submissives is so skewed, it's that you're slowly weeding out dominants who you can tell right from the start will not fit your needs, which, by its nature cuts your working field by a significant margin.

When searching for a dominant, you are not looking for just anyone who proclaims themselves to be a dominant. You're seeking the Yin to your Yang, the dominant who likes what you like, complements you as much as you compliment them, and making sure you're both at the same level of "intensity." By intensity I mean if you like to be lightly spanked and they like to take out an intense wooden paddle – there may be an incompatibility when it comes to the intensity of 'play' which could very easily create a problem. If one of you loves needle-play while the other considers anything sharp and shiny (or blood related) to be a hard limit, there are going to be frustrations within the relationship or play-partnership. I'm trying to avoid saying "skill level" because having an interest in something does not equate to skill.

Most importantly, you are not looking for a dominant who will accept you as their submissive and then will make you change every single thing about you, including your desires, just to be with you. **No!!!** This is a terrible idea and if this is how you're thinking about finding a dominant not only will you likely fail and/or piss off dominants along the way; but you will also find yourself incredibly miserable as your own needs are not going to be met. This wastes everyone's time, generates hard feelings, and may even discourage you from wanting to search again. I do want to say, however, there are those who do lean towards the more extreme aspects of the lifestyle who do seek significant changes in their life (and even their bodies or minds) but that's a book for another day. Let's stay focused on the basics for now.

Being a submissive does not mean losing your identity

Do not confuse submissive and slave (read the chapters discussing specific terms). Again, as I mentioned, there are some very, very, very select few "slaves" who do want to hand over their entire life, well-being, and even their identity to an owner. However, as a submissive, you typically want to retain some of your own "self" and find someone with whom you can build a mutually beneficial relationship, regardless of the relationship dynamic. That means you give and take and they take and give – to what extent, and on what terms, is up to both of you to **agree** upon as being acceptable. Some changes, adaptations, and continued education are a requirement but remember...

Never, ever lose your "self"

SECTION ONE:
UNDERSTANDING DEFINITIONS

Perhaps one of the biggest problems in searching for
"the one" is a rampant misunderstanding of terminology.
*Clarifying and understanding what **you** are and knowing in clear terms*
what you are seeking will help save a lot of time and hard feelings.

Chapter 1

What Are You?

There's the unfortunate fact that terms such as **slave** and **submissive** are used equally and rather interchangeably despite having different meanings. In fact, they're not the only terms one can use to identify in this lifestyle. Some of the first steps before ever considering contact with a dominant are to discover how you identify, how you fit into those labels, and how to clearly inform others of how you are identifying. The latter is most important since labels can be interpreted in a variety of ways and people can "kind of" fit into one while also fitting into another. Some people may have two completely different views for the exact same label. So clarification is important.

Of course, this isn't necessarily an all-encompassing list since ways to self-identify are always changing and evolving. Trying to fit into one tidy neat box, especially in this lifestyle, is like forcing a square object into a circular hole. Do not feel like you must pick a label or force yourself to fit into a label, but if you feel a connection with one then you should understand it and know how to express yourself within that context so dominants can get a better understanding of you, what you're seeking, and if that is in alignment with what they're seeking.

My purpose here is to provide some basic understanding and guidance on what the terminology means and how those terms are interpreted. If you list that you're a slave but you're really a fetishist chances are you're going to:

- Email the wrong people who aren't going to be able to fulfill your desires.

- Get no response because you're not presenting yourself correctly or well.

- Ruin the chance of, at the very least, gaining a friend or guide who could refer you to the "one true goddess" of your dreams.

I'll stop here for a moment to put in a brief disclaimer. If there's one truth in this lifestyle, perhaps more so than anywhere else, it is that "terms" and "labels" are almost never all-encompassing or binding. Definitions will vary from person to person to include or exclude certain nuances. They will vary depending on who you are with, what you do and don't like, and where you are at this moment in your life. Understanding the general concept of each term will help you focus your search but shouldn't be thought of as the end-all-be-all of 'who' you are. It is your responsibility to define and refine your interpretation of the label(s) you use in your profile or to briefly explain it when emailing a dominant so you can ask if it matches or is close to the dominant's impression of the term.

Important Disclaimer: As I mentioned previously, there's truly no one way to define yourself or someone else. Not only can you claim multiple labels but many of the terms blend and bleed into each other. In the instances of cross-dressing and sissification or feminization, many use the terms interchangeably while others will separate them as wholly different. It could make one's head explode trying to pin down clear lines and definitions but one aspect that many love about our lifestyle is that we're not boxed in by typical societal restrictions and expectations. Why restrict yourself within the lifestyle that's meant to give us freedom? This is merely an attempt to provide a broad or basic understanding of the more commonly used terms that you can then use as an aid in some self-discovery. You won't want to contact a dominant who feels that forced feminization is insulting while you find it as a necessary part of play, nor would you want to contact a dominant for pet-play who hates it or just doesn't understand or have interest in it. Luckily, many of these fetishes, desires, and interests have innumerable groups and websites dedicated to them (not just porn) to help you narrow down your interests. But first, let's understand what some of them mean.

Common Terms

Headspace: This is a term that you will hear quite often and it can sometimes be interchanged with "sub-space" (which we will discuss in a later chapter). The two terms are a bit different so in this regard, I am referring to the state of mind of fully embracing the level of submission or role that you're attempting to realize. Some are content with a subtle feeling while others seek total immersion. This could be something you experience or bring yourself to for just a scene or something you seek to be your way of thinking for your life.

24/7: This is a common reference used and is pretty self-explanatory. It simply means all day every day. Sometimes it includes the bit redundant addition of 365 (24/7/365) to include "all year." It's frequently used to indicate the person wants something "all the time" or "without break." Essentially, a permanent arrangement rather than just play partners.

Slave: There is much debate about what this term actually means and how it can be applied both legally and within the lifestyle. This "definition" is my own personal take on the matter and it comes from the perspective that I live an M/s lifestyle rather than a more well-known D/s one in conjunction with substantial research into the subject matter.

In general, a slave is someone who is prepared to give over all their rights, decision making, possessions, and entire being to an owner. The little intricacies on how your owner can/will make you feel like a slave is up to you and the owner to whom you eventually surrender. Those who dedicate themselves to the Master/slave (M/s) lifestyle are often looked down upon in the lifestyle because it is "too extreme" or far too likely to be exploited by those with malicious intent.

Stating that you are a slave is asserting that you are looking for an extremely intense, hard-core, all-inclusive situation and is often referred to online as a TPE (Total Power Exchange). This often, by default, means you're looking for a 24/7, live-in relationship albeit there is the sub-category of 'slave role-play,' which I'll discuss next. There are plenty of owners out there who are seeking slaves but there are also plenty of dominants who see "slave" and don't want to go anywhere near that type of lifestyle.

Slave Role-Play: Role-playing is, in itself, a popular activity within the lifestyle and will be discussed on its own. However, I want to briefly cover the 'slave role-play' as previously mentioned. To be a slave inherently implies a 24/7 live-in dynamic but, as with anything in life, too much of something can either become overwhelming or, at the very least, stale. Some may be madly in love with the Master/slave (M/s) concept but for whatever reasons are unable to incorporate that into their daily lives. In role-play a solution can be found for many forms of expression and slavery is certainly one of them.

Slavery in a role-play setting requires just as much negotiation and understanding but can include pretending to be anything, from being an actualized present-day slave to being a slave from the Roman Empire or any other era your heart desires. The major difference is that after a pre-set amount of time the "fantasy" ends and you both return to your regular lives/dynamic.

Submissive/s-type: This is perhaps one of the most common terms in the lifestyle and is used for nearly everyone looking to serve, regardless of intensity or capacity. It's lost the clarity of its definition over the years but there are still many out there who take the term for what it means.

A submissive is looking for a kind of power exchange dynamic, which runs the gamut from living in an otherwise "vanilla" relationship with a little D/s thrown in for spice to engaging in a 24/7 lifestyle. Typically, there is an equal amount of giving and taking in this relationship and the manner of expressing submission is also widely varied.

A submissive can be someone who enjoys the act of submitting to others regardless of gender or to only the one who may hold their collar. That is to say, this person will show submissive qualities to all dominants as a sign of respect and as a way to fulfill their pleasure in submission or, alternatively, will see all others as their equal except their owner/dominant who is the only one privy to receive their acts of submission. Some are submissive to any dominant but of only one gender while others have no gender restrictions. Despite showing respect, it is important for both the submissive and dominant to remember: "they may be submissive, but they are not *your* submissive." Many submissives will cite this when they feel a dominant is not respecting boundaries with a submissive person who is not their own submissive.

It's important not to equate submission with weakness nor to think that just because someone is a dominant they are somehow above showing basic respect and common courtesy to others, submissives included. If a dominant brings a submissive a drink because they happened to be up at the time, it does not mean they're an inadequate dominant but merely that they're being a courteous human. Just because a submissive grabs a dominant a plate of snacks doesn't mean they're surrendering themselves to that (or any other) dominant, but merely just being attentive and helpful to someone who happens to be a dominant person. You will see s-type most often as a quick form of submissive such as in chats or groups.

Bottom: This is someone who really isn't interested in serving or submitting but likes to 'bottom' to certain activities (such as a kink discussed a little further down). It's usually a matter of having something done to you rather than you serving/submitting to a dominant (or, in this case, a top) in order to achieve your desires. A top who loves to spank asses would match up with a bottom who loves OTK (Over The Knee spanking). Many view those not interested in servitude as a bottom. Once again, this isn't the 'absolute' when it comes to definitions but by and large, a bottom is either looking to be the physical bottom (or non-aggressor) in a sexual encounter or the receiver of a kinky action with little to no expectation of actual submission outside of that specific context.

Role-Play Terms

I want to preface this specific section of terms by stating that there are genuine submissives who truly love, enjoy, and even crave brattiness, sissification, age-play, and pet-play. They and their dominants have found ways to incorporate these desires into their lives, but they are often secondary to the overall D/s dynamic. There are also those who seek to engage only in this type of behavior without submission being a factor or these acts are their form of submission.

Role-Play: This is a more all-encompassing term for those interested in engaging in scenes or play that take them out of their everyday 'headspace' and put them into a specific mindset, as discussed previously with slaves. However, becoming a weekend slave is not the only role-play available. It could be Priest/Nun, Captor(Interrogator)/Prisoner, or any other pairing your imagination can conjure. It can also include dominant and submissive for those who just enjoy a little touch of spice in their life during specific "play/scenes" but otherwise have an equal relationship dynamic.

Brats: Those who enjoy doing things, on purpose, to egg their dominant on or to get a specific reaction from their dominant. Many say this is topping from the bottom while others just call them brats. Because the "submissive" is essentially "asking for it" by purposefully disobeying or misbehaving in some way, many don't see this as submission at all. It can, however, be incorporated as role-playing where the "submissive" can better embrace or get through a scene, discipline, or other D/s type activities only when they are expressing their brattiness. Some dominants like the tug and pull and the sense of being kept alert and "on their toes" that a brat can provide, rather than a more – in some ways – monotonous routine.

Littles/Middles: Those who enjoy either regressing to a younger age or at least partaking in dress or behaviors of a younger age. This can range from just being called "baby girl/boy" to dressing and acting the age they desire, to full-blown mental regression to the age they want to inhabit. This is also called age-play, little-play, or infant-play. Mommy(Daddy)/baby girl(boy) is a fairly common aspect of the lifestyle and is often just one portion of their D/s lives expressed in ways as varied as enjoying some quiet time coloring to wearing diapers and all the accouterments of a baby/toddler. This can be enjoyed with the subtly of a Daddy/Mommy providing their little with the coloring menu at a restaurant to full-blown littles-based events and gatherings. There are, unfortunately, a few too many people within the general lifestyle who shun or misunderstand these interests so there are those who are hesitant to express their desires in this regard.

Pets: These truly run the spectrum of the animal kingdom from puppy/dog, kitten/cat, to wolves, pigs, or all other types of animals.

There are two primary areas of identification within this subset, the first is described as, or called, **"feral-play"** as it ultimately allows those involved to sink into their most primal of headspaces. This can be very cathartic but also dangerous, as most people revert to their baser, or primal, instincts. The second and more common variety is **"pet-play"** and refers to the taking on of animal characteristics and even immersing oneself into the mindset of the chosen animal. Many find this as a way to express a primitive level of their submission such as a dog submits to its master, or how a beta wolf submits to its alpha. Others feel they share a deep kinship with the chosen animal and wish to embody it while others just enjoy the subjugation of being treated as just an animal. This may include being led by collar and leash, fed scraps from the table, eating/drinking from pet bowls, and crawling on all-fours. Others enjoy playful acts like playing fetch, belly rubs, and just curling up in a pet bed. Often when a person is in their pet-play mindset, regardless of the animal chosen, they do not speak but use the ways in which that animal may communicate such as yips, barks, meows, growls, oinks, and so forth. Sometimes they and their owner develop a specific way that certain "sounds" or inflections of that sound will convey specific things although often it's easy enough to decipher the overall intention of the sounds given the body language and inflections much as we would with traditional animals.

Furries: While this is not a kink it is often misunderstood and often lumped into the world of kink. While furries can be in the lifestyle and can express their furry-ness within the lifestyle, the actual interest or identification of being a furry is not a kink. They often refer to themselves as a fandom which celebrates a wide variety of interests/fandoms and often has nothing to do with sex or kink. There is, of course, a subset within the furries who do enjoy a sexualized aspect of being furry and, again, the two lifestyles can overlap but that is only because of the specific individuals and not that one group (kink/lifestyle) or another (furry) are of the same ilk.

Pony-Play: I am separating this entirely from the pet-play category because it is an entity unto itself. There are events, lifestyles, facilities, and even industries designed specifically to cater to pony play. This is much as it sounds – people who wish to dress and or submerge themselves into the mindset (again, to varying degrees) of being a ponyboy/ponygirl and engage with Trainers. Pony-play can become integral parts of their lives, spending small fortunes on outfits/gear (tack), saddles or rigging that accommodate riding a human pony, carts (or sulkies) for ponies to pull, and detailed head and foot gear that emulate a horse. As with other pets/animals, when in the mindset of a pony they will not speak and will often only respond with a nod or shake of the head, a stomp of the feet, or a whinny. Just as with real horses some can be a bit spirited or playful while others strictly follow the direction of their trainer.

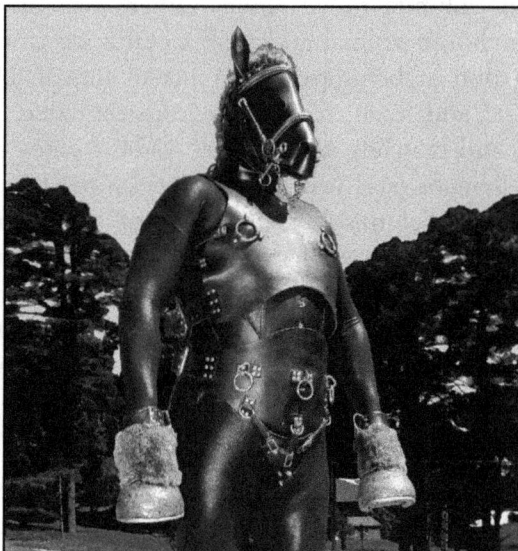

Photo credit to Tigger, used with permission.

Gender-Related Terms

Sissies: Males who enjoy, either of on their own accord or by being made by another, to dress in women's clothing. Envision a male in a maid's uniform. While a popular fantasy, it is not the only way to experience this desire. Many males have a sissification fetish and there are plenty of dominants who enjoy and embrace this. Others will use the threat (and the actual following-through) of, sissification as a form of punishment or humiliation (especially where humiliation is also a fetish). However, degradation does not have to be a factor, as sissification can be something that a male just truly enjoys, whether it's the sensation of the fabrics against his skin or the mental state it helps him find while wearing panties, women's shoes, or other women-designated items.

Note of Caution: Some people may find a male's interest in sissification/ feminization to be insulting if done because the male feels it will humiliate him to be treated like a female. They may feel that because – essentially – the male is saying a woman is weak, undesirable, and inherently less-than. This is especially a more sensitive issue more recently and those who are interested in sissification/ forced-feminization should acquaint themselves with what's happening in the world presently with women and the overall inequality they face and come at this fetish with at least some kind of respect. This is not to say that dominants, even FemDoms, do not enjoy sissification/feminization of men as many find it equally thrilling as the men do, but it won't hurt to just be aware of the current climate.

Cross-Dresser (CD): Once again we tread into murky waters in the sense that there's a lot of mixing and mingling of terms, but some people make a clear delineation between sissy and CD. That demarcation would be that a cross-dresser identifies as the opposite gender, whether for events-only, in private-only, or on a full-time basis, but does not necessarily identify as a transgender person nor do they seek to actually transition. They are satiated with dressing the part and taking on some (or all) of the mannerisms without relinquishing the gender in which they were assigned at birth. While it's most often equated with men seeking to dress in clothing typically associated with women, there are women who enjoy dressing in what is often equated with men. This could include wearing suits, men's underwear/jocks, or other "masculine" clothing.

Drag Queen/King: Being a Drag Queen has become incredibly public and popular thanks to *RuPaul's Drag Race* and associated spin-offs (2009 - present). Drag has been around nearly as long as people have and there are amazing historical accounts of women dressing in drag in order to fight in wars and other truly interesting aspects of drag-history that are beyond the scope of this book but definitely worth investigating further. Often not considered but equally important are the Drag Kings. Without going into a dissertation on drag, suffice it to say that a Drag Queen/King is someone who dresses as the opposite gender (in which they were assigned at birth) but do so with the intent to entertain. While Drag Kings tend to dress in a manner to be most in-line with the typical male look, Drag Queens often dress in a manner that is an exaggeration of women frequently to glamorous effect. In most cases a drag person does not identify as the gender they are representing and are happy to live their lives as a cis-gender person and consider drag to be a performance and a character in which to embody for just a period of time. That's not to say that some drag people eventually transition because they've discovered they were transgender through their work in drag, but drag and transgender are not the same things. Additionally, while drag can be incorporated into the lifestyle, like most other things it is not considered a kink or fetish.

Transgender: The transgender community is a complex matter and, as such, will be covered in its own chapter. The quick takeaway is that trans people are not fetishes, are not role-playing, and are frequently misunderstood and misrepresented. Whether you are interested in transgender people or not you will likely encounter a trans person in your life, especially in this lifestyle, so read the chapter to avoid issues and stop ongoing ignorance.

Fetish Terms

Fetishist: While many of the aforementioned terms can easily fit here as well, I wanted to separate them on purpose. If you have a passion for a specific thing, but otherwise don't really want to submit or serve, you are a fetishist. That is to say, if you love how latex feels and your wardrobe for a night out consists of a great deal of it then you may be a fetishist. Fetishes and kinks are other examples of terms being used interchangeably yet having two distinct meanings. If your sexual desire and pleasure are derived from an object (i.e. latex, shoes, panties, etc.) that is a fetish. As such, you are a fetishist if that specific thing is the necessary center and focus of your play, scenes, or exchanges. This is not to say that you cannot be dominant or submissive while also being a fetishist, but if your goals are to engage in fetish-based activities rather than serving then designating yourself as a fetishist will help pinpoint your searches. Fetishes can be and often are key elements in a D/s dynamic, but they are incorporated into the dynamic that is still, at its foundation, built on the exchange of dominance and submission. If you are not that interested in submitting to someone or will only submit under the terms of having that specific fetish being explored then you're more a fetishist than a submissive.

Kinkster: While a fetishist derives sexual pleasure from an object, Kink itself is defined as engaging in an activity and deriving your pleasure, desire, and/or lust from doing this activity. This does not default to mean that enjoying a certain kink means you want to submit. It means you want to engage in this particular activity – usually as a top or a bottom . For example, you enjoy being spanked over someone's knee (OTK) but once you're upright you're not expected to submit or serve. This is how many "weekend warriors" or those looking for a little spice in the bedroom, would most likely find themselves. You can enjoy being a kinkster and serving at the same time but, again, if your primary mission is to explore your kinks with little expectation of submission or serving outside of the scene then you are better off by clarifying yourself as a Kinkster.

Masochist: This is someone for whom fetish, kink, service, submission and all else fall secondary to pain, someone who actively seeks out pain as they receive the most pleasure and intense enjoyment from that pain. There are, of course, varying levels of pain tolerance and very different tastes in the causes of the pain, but it boils down to being a **pain slut** (a very common term for a masochist). Pain releases endorphins and many thrive on the rush this creates. In the vanilla world they may be "Thrill Seekers" or "Adrenaline Junkies" but in the BDSM lifestyle, they're called masochists because they derive the same sense of exhilaration from the infliction of pain. While one masochist may thrive on whips and other 'stinging' sensations another masochist may not be able to handle (or process the pain) from that kind of implement but may instead favor blunted instruments like paddles. Just because a masochist thrives on pain doesn't mean all pain is the same. It was previously diagnosed (along with many of the other 'acts' in our lifestyle) as a mental disorder but was redefined in the DSM-IV 2000 revision.

As an aside: The lifestyle exists on its own covenant of Safe, Sane, and Consensual (SSC) which is typically the basic foundation for anyone in the lifestyle. There are those who also practice Risk Aware Consensual Kink (RACK) which tends to be what those use to identify they are into more "edgy" aspects of the lifestyle. Regardless, the community as a whole does tend to police itself and takes the overall safety of the members and community with great seriousness. They will not let one person/couple/household bring ruin to the greater community. Those who pose a risk by unsafe play, non-consensual acts, or out-right illegal acts could be banned from events/spaces or even turned over to the police. Play safe and within the confines of consent (even non-consensual consent) and everyone will have a good time. Break the tenet of the lifestyle and you will not be welcome.

Not Terms of Endearment

These terms are often used as an insult or in some derogatory manner. While some might be used endearingly between dominant and submissive, it's usually rare and typically one wants to avoid being referred to by any of the following terms.

Smart Ass Masochist (SAM): This is someone who is often a brat, but will engage in teasing (bratty) behavior not only to be playful or to keep a dominant on their toes but typically do so with the express purpose of egging a dominant into a response, even if it means being 'punished' for bad behavior – as long as it gets them attention and the treatment they're seeking. Sometimes this is done playfully, but can also come off as really snarky, disrespectful, or just outright rude. It is up to the individual dominant on how they choose to respond to a SAM – engage in the scene/play or ignore the behavior.

Do-Me Sub/Bottom: This attitude is also among the top pet peeves of dominants. These submissives or bottoms will do whatever they can (flattery or inciting) to provoke a dominant to scene with them or do something specific to/for the Do-Me Sub/Bottom and then they're simply done and walk away. They have no follow-through, no intention of submission or service, and sometimes can even be disinterested in ensuring the dominant/top is satiated. Sometimes they will do only the minimal act of submission but still only with the intent of getting only what they want from the dominant.

As you can see, there are many ways for you to identify yourself and, within each of those labels, there are infinite gradations to further define or clarify your chosen role. Everyone is different with a different kink or spin on their desires and the definitions above can be broadened or shortened to fit.

You can see how defining yourself as one thing can be very misleading if it's not what you truly mean. Many newbies pick a label because they like the "sound" of it with very little real understanding of what it means or entails. If you're a fetishist, but picked the title "slave" and you start emailing owners, it is an effort in futility. You're wasting your time and theirs because eventually (and usually it doesn't take too long if either of you has been around enough) one or both of you will discover this is not the right match and end the whole process, sometimes bitterly.

By understanding that you're a kinkster, you can email those who seem to be as well, so you can try to develop a connection and let it grow from there. Misunderstanding labels and where people can fit within them means you will wind up not just wasting everyone's time and energies, but you could easily develop a bad reputation. People do share this kind of information online and in real life communities to warn of potential "trolls."

Even if you enjoy scrolling random profiles, once you know what you are and what you're looking for, you can "search" the website and quickly eliminate the non-starters so you can pinpoint the potentials and spend your time (and theirs) more wisely. It also helps cut down on the rejections. Enough rejections (or non-answers) can easily cause a person to become dejected enough to just give up entirely. It's hard enough making a match when you're all in the same interest group because of chemistry and other factors, but spreading yourself so thin because you're looking in the wrong place can make many just throw up their hands. You're left, now, being completely unsated as a person and a kinkster but could also develop a bad taste in your mouth for the lifestyle as a whole which would be a shame. The lifestyle is an amazing place, once you find your niche.

To avoid this, it may mean spending time actually reading, not just this book, but other resources (there are plenty online) that will help you further understand what you are, where your interests lie, and how to identify the profiles of dominants who share your interests.

Access the Internet and its infinite resources (including those listed at the end of this book) but take everything you find with a grain of salt. Remember, when it comes to labels it really boils down to personal interpretation and how it fits into their own life. Take from each of the definitions what you will and incorporate what you can. Just know, the more you understand what each term means and can narrow down what you, in turn, are seeking, the better shot you have of finding that elusive dominant. That is the ultimate goal – finding your match so you can have the fulfillment you seek. If you're going to spend the time and make the effort, do it the best way possible.

Chapter 2

What Are They?

Everything in life has its opposite; the Yin to the Yang; the Heads to the Tails… you get the point, so obviously, there is the dominant to the submissive. Common sense would lead you to believe many of the terms discussed in the previous chapter have their companion although sometimes specific opposites are limited. That is to say, while a submissive-type can identify as a brat, there's no specific term for a dominant that likes bratty behavior. Unless they include 'Dominant who loves brats' in their profile you are left without much of a clue that this is something they may enjoy. For the other labels that do have counterparts, I will break them down and discuss them here.

It is important for you to recognize how the dominant has chosen to identify so as to avoid confusion or simply not to go barking up the wrong tree. Many dominants (like most people in general) take great care in selecting how they identify, whether because the identifier (or attached honorific) is important to them or because they simply want to weed out the riff-raff. There are also plenty of dominants who are new or just don't care and will select random titles or labels just because it sounds sexy or "dominating" to them with little care to the genuine meaning or the responsibilities typically associated with that label.

Common Terms

First and Foremost:

Whether you're a dominant or a submissive it's imperative to understand the difference between **Dominant** and **Dominate**. You cannot **BE** a *dominate*. Dominant (in this instance) is the noun and thus is the 'title.' Dominate is the action, it is the thing a dominant does to the submissive. This is a huge peeve among many in the lifestyle and having this wrong in your profile (whether you're dominant or submissive) will instantly turn most people off from any further consideration.

FemDom: Often mistaken or assumed to be a dominant who is feminine. However, the term strictly means a dominant who is female and that means anyone who identifies as female. Additionally, it's important to remember that women come in all shapes, sizes, ethnicities, backgrounds, and so forth. Do not assume FemDom means a tall, svelte, leather-clad strict-looking cis woman who is all too often depicted in pornography because that's not the reality. While those women do exist they're not the only FemDoms and female dominants run an amazing gamut of physical appearances and personalities. So, simply put, FemDom is Female Dominant.

Male Dominant: There really is no specification for "male dominant" as there is for FemDom. However, I want to point out that there is a general misleading image of what a male dominant should look/be like at times and people need to remember that male dominants also come in every incarnation of appearance and personality.

Dominants D-type: Dominants do not dominate every second of their lives. While many have a naturally dominant presence or "way about them," most are generally laid-back and, just like anyone else, live their daily lives, but can exude seductive domination when so inclined. Some are not dominant except within the context of a scene or an established role-play. There also seems to be a misconception that domination is the same thing as or needs to have "meanness" involved. Some of the most "badass" dominants I've ever known were calm, soft-spoken, and very polite to everyone, but they can dominate, control a scene, wield an implement, or push someone into a headspace like a boss. You may see D-type used mainly in chat rooms or groups as it's a lot easier and faster to write that than constantly spell out dominants.

Headspace: Dominants reach their own headspace and often feed off the actions and reactions of their partner, enhancing the experience for the submissive and creating a fulfilling energy cycle.

That is to say – the more submissive acting the submissive is, the more engrossed the dominant becomes in their domineering headspace, which then, in turn, promotes more submission from the submissive.

Owner: This can be used for two different subsets of the lifestyle. The first being for those interested in the M/s (Master/slave) lifestyle arrangement. While Master and Mistress or other honorifics can all equally be used, many will at least include in their profile that they are an "owner" to help differentiate that they are specifically into M/s. The other is used by those who are into pet-play dynamics in the sense of being a pet owner. Again, other titles/honorifics can be used but an all-encompassing term for tops/dominants into pet-play could be Owner.

Mistress/Domina/Domme: These are extremely common titles that are pretty much all-encompassing. Professionals will take on these titles for simplicity sake but, unfortunately, there's little way to determine what the dominant is into simply by title alone, other than the fact they identify in some capacity as a dominant. While many will use just this term throughout their entire interaction with submissives (or the community in general), some will use them just for a scene or an event and some will have only their own submissive use these honorifics while others can use something like Miss (see below).

Ma'am/Miss/Ms.: Many dominants have taken on honorifics of this nature. While it may appear to have a "softer" sense than Mistress do not make the mistake of assuming they are any less domineering as someone else with a more strict title. These can also be used as alternatives for a submissive to use while in more public spaces or during less formal instances of service (such as daily service as opposed to a play party/event).

Female Masters/Sirs: While not overly common there are females who opt for "masculine" titles. This could be for any number of reasons and I have personally known very feminine women who use Master. Paying attention to profiles (discussed in detail later) is important. Not every woman wants to be called Mistress and perhaps not every Master/Sir you see is a man. Pay attention to how the person gender identifies.

Goddess/Lady/Ultra Femme Terms: These titles will give you a small clue into the personality of those who choose them. They tell a prospective submissive that the dominant is highly feminine. While I'm not saying those who select any other title don't like to be ultra-femme, as many do, but when a dominant opts for a title along these lines you can tell almost instantly you're dealing with a DivaDom. And I don't mean Diva in a bad, overly dramatic way by any means.

Sirs: A common title for dominants (as discussed it can be for any gender identification although it is most commonly associated with those who identify as male). This can be the only title which a dominant uses or it could be similar to that of Miss/Ma'am wherein the dominant will use another title (like Master) but will use Sir in more public spaces. This is also a good default for submissives to use when not sure how the dominant may wish to be addressed. Additionally, some may opt for **Lord** or similar titles.

Master: While this is typically seen as the counterpart to Mistress this title often gets a lot of backlash. To "master" something typically means that you've dedicated a large part of your time and efforts to something and are incredibly skilled. When someone (typically) under 30 years old, but especially 25 years and younger, uses this title it will often be scoffed or at the very least receive an eye-roll. While anyone is free to use whatever title they want, I would recommend exercising some caution of younger people throwing this title around. That being said, this is a fairly common honorific used by dominants.

Top: This is someone who enjoys taking the lead in situations, physically being on top, or otherwise taking the more aggressive role but doesn't necessarily want to be dominant. Their counterpoint is the bottom.

Role-Play Terms

Bigs/Mommy/Daddy: These are the counterparts to littles/middles and the terms Mommy and Daddy can be used regardless of gender as the roles are entirely dependent on how the dominant identifies. The Big (as Mommy/Daddy types are referred to collectively) will play a parent-like role to the little most often with play/games, but will periodically provide discipline as a parent would to a child but more in line with the mentality. That is, if a little got into trouble they wouldn't get a flogging necessarily but may get corner time or a spanking such as Over The Knee (OTK). When dealing with a little but especially one who regresses, the Big must ensure a mentally and physically safe space as many littles/middles are vulnerable while immersed in that headspace.

(Pet) Owners: These people will behave much like typical pet owners. They will stroke (pet) their "pets" hair, will hand-feed scraps, or put food in bowls, play fetch with their dog/puppy or turn a laser light on to tease their kitten/cat.

When speaking to their submissive who is fully engrossed in their animal-self, they will often limit the conversation to things one would say to a pet, like "go fetch." Some pets will just take on characteristics of the animal they like, so the owners can engage in a more 'human-like manner.'

Trainers: This most often references those who handle ponies. A trainer is responsible for their pony, whether teaching them dressage, working them in the lunging ring, or having them pull carts. This means ensuring that their pony gets carrots or apples to eat, plenty of water, and proper grooming. As there is a great deal of pony gear available, many trainers will dress the part as well, donning outfits that you'd see at riding academies or derbies.

Gender-Related Terms

Just as there are men who prefer to dress or take on the likeness or role of a woman there are many women who will take on the persona of men. This could be limited to role-playing during sexual activities or involve much more of their lives.

Cross Dressers: Some FemDoms enjoy wearing the clothing or taking on the style of a man. She may wear leather pants and a vest in lieu of a corset and a skirt. There is typically a more masculine aspect to her, perhaps a subtle way of carrying herself or more overt attempts to alter her body language in a manly way. Being a crossdresser does not automatically mean the dominant is a lesbian or even that she identifies as being transgender, merely that she feels fulfilled and most comfortable when dressed as a male whether it's just for that scene or for everything else. I've yet to encounter a scenario where a male dominant cross dresses but that is not to say it never happens and, therein, is something to just be mindful of as a possibility.

Transgender: As noted in Chapter 1 there is a chapter dedicated to the TGNC community.

Fetish Terms

Fetishist/Kinkster: Yes, these terms apply to dominants as well. This is a person who enjoys dressing in fetish-ware such as leather or latex. Perhaps a dominant with their own foot fetish in the form of having their feet sucked/licked. They are someone who is more interested in exploring specific aspects of a kink without necessarily taking on a full-time dominant role.

Sadist: A sadist complements the masochist by being the one who derives pleasure from giving another person pain. The methods of applying that pain can vary drastically but ultimately the sadist is someone who is good at delivering the pain and knows what they are doing to ensure safe play. Someone who just beats on another or uses the tools of our lifestyle with reckless abandon are NOT sadists. They're either ignorant people who think they know what they're doing and are greatly mistaken or they're abusers using the guise of being a sadist (or dominant in general) to get away with it. Remember, play safe and smart, even if you both strive for pain.

Professional/Pro-Dom/me/Dominatrix: (Note: FinDom is different) Professional Dom/mes have suffered a bad rap and it's mostly due to the

Internet and specifically because of FinDoms. Primarily professionals are female but there are the occasional professional male dominants. Because of the ease and anonymity of the web, many have taken advantage of it, and its users, to sucker folks into sending money and gifts under the guise of being a "Pro Dom" when, in reality, they're just scam artists (more on scams in Chapter 5).

To the vanilla world, professionals are little more than prostitutes, whether they engage in sexual acts or not doesn't seem to matter. While it's okay to hire a contractor to come to my home, perform their specialized service and pay them for their time, it is not okay (in the eyes of many) to pay a professional dominant who is skilled in domination to provide that service for compensation.

Without getting into an entire historical perspective of professional domination or an analytical debate on "Professional Dominant versus Prostitute" I'll focus on genuine Pro-Dom/mes. They have honed their skills and have built their abilities through years being **active** in the lifestyle and are comfortable and proficient performing a variety of BDSM related scenes and activities.

Furthermore, this is someone who asks important questions, takes your hard limits seriously, and cares about your mental and physical safety before, during, and after a session. They know what to do in an emergency and have a vast array of skills to offer. If you go to a professional and they want to know your limits and ask you medical/ safety questions this is often a good indicator that they have some experience. Also any professional worth their salt will offer references from those around the community from both submissives and dominants.

There is no regulation or licensing with professional dominants. There are also far too many fakes out there that have inundated the various sites. If you're interested in a genuine professional ask around in your local community. If it's a nameless/faceless Internet being it's better to avoid them altogether.

FinDom: This is non-gender specific and is the more appropriate term to use for those who seek to just scam others or for those who specifically love to be taken advantage of especially when it comes to money. This is, specifically, Financial Domination. Whether it's something both parties agree on or they manage to dup the submissive, the end is typically little to no real contact with the "dominant" and will often consist of being spoken to in a way that gets the "submissive" hot and bothered and then shown images of the "dominant" that are often stolen from across the web. In "exchange" for the attention, the "dominant" has shown the "submissive" they must now pay and typically by means of a variety of services that will allow for anonymous access on the FinDom's part. This could also include sending them gifts off their wish lists from all kinds of websites. Either way, the submissive pays out financially and often gets nothing but a fantasy screw as a result.

Chapter 3

What Is That?

General Terms

LGBT+: This is also called the Alphabet Soup at times considering how extended it's becoming. You may see examples be as extensive as LGBTQQIP2SAA which stands for Lesbian, Gay, Bisexual, Transgender, Queer, Questioning, Intersex, Pansexual, 2-spirited, Asexual, and Allies. In many cases, it's shortened to LGBT+ to make it still a manageable acronym but with the + acting as an acknowledgment to all the other gender identities and sexualities as even the most extended version doesn't cover all. It's a good thing to get in the habit of including the + whenever you write LGBT otherwise you may get called out for it being too limited or not acknowledging the large scopes of gender and sexuality.

BDSM: Most assume it just means Bondage Discipline Sadomasochism but the D and S are doing double duty. It's more appropriately broken down as Bondage & Discipline – Dominance & Submission – Sadism & Masochism.

Switch: This is someone who enjoys being both submissive and dominant depending on how they feel that day or depending on the type of partner (or even gender) with whom they engage. Some women will be dominant with men but will submit to women or vice versa. Some want to find a partner who is also a switch so they can each take on the different roles whenever they want. Others will switch only under certain circumstances.

Just like most other things in this lifestyle, there's plenty of ways to enjoy being a switch but the bottom line is, this person enjoys taking on either role so this is something to consider. Do you want a dominant who will only be dominant with you but it's okay if they are submissive to someone else at the same time or under certain circumstances or do you want a dominant who is only dominant? If you're fine with the person being a switch as long as they are dominant with you or if you think you're a switch as well and would like to explore with other switches, be sure to read their profiles carefully as they will often explain under what conditions in which they will switch.

Poly/Non-Monogamy: Scientists are discovering that non-monogamy is common among many species and while it's often considered in a negative way polyamory can be an incredibly fulfilling relationship. We've seen some aspects of this peeking its way into the mainstream with some shows and movies using the term "throuple" to indicate a three-way relationship, which is one way to engage in a poly dynamic. The myriad ways in which these dynamics can be explored is extensive and there are books dedicated solely to this topic. The main thing is to just be aware that relationships aren't always between two people and can be engaged in many different ways with a variety of partners in a slew of dynamics. Also, know that this type of relationship dynamic can be very difficult to navigate and requires trust and constantly open avenues of communication.

To Out/Outing: This is something that no one should do to anyone else in any capacity in any facet of their lives. This is especially dangerous when you out someone who is LGBT+ as it's still legal in most of the United States for someone to be fired, have adoptions declined, be excommunicated, and otherwise denied basic civil liberties based solely on their sexuality or gender identity. It could also result in gay-bashing or death.

To out someone as being within the BDSM community in any capacity could be equally dangerous, and while it rarely results in being physically attacked or murdered because the person is found to be kinky they can still lose their jobs, lose their families, have their children taken away, and any other number of devastating life-altering impacts. Even if the person seems 100% at ease with their kinkiness and even if they do things that seem "obviously kinky" to you while out in vanilla circumstances it is NEVER, EVER, NEVER, EVER, NEVER EVER acceptable to out anyone in any way. End of story! The community does NOT take kindly to those who out others and will often close ranks and expel the person who has outed someone. If they cannot expel the person they will treat the outing person with distance and will not invite them to things whenever possible.

This can be done in a million ways and most often the person who is doing the outing doesn't even realize they've done it so outing someone doesn't have to be with malicious intent. Be extremely conscious of what you say about others and to whom you speak.

Giving someone a "preface" is also a form of outing them. Unless you're at a kink event or things have been discussed previously and agreed upon by both persons, never say things in a general vanilla setting like: "This is John Smith, he's a submissive," or "This is my slave, Jane Doe." It is rare that a slip like this would happen but what does happen with alarming regularity is LGBT+ prefacing. Things like: "This is my gay friend, John," or "This is my trans friend, Jude." Not only is it rude to do since you should be speaking to and about people like you would anyone else, but it's also incredibly dangerous and absolutely not tolerated.

FOR EXAMPLE:

There was a person who was a member of one of the local communities in which I was also involved. While I am generally extremely open about my sexuality and gender identity, I am well aware of when within certain instances it's better to just not say anything at all as I live always having this as a thought. However, the white, straight, male person who has never had to live with any concerns about someone finding his mere presence threatening or an abomination saw no issues with announcing to non-lifestyle friends that I was lesbian or that I was transitioning, or that I was once a female. Given that we were in the south it was entirely possible that any one of those people could have attacked me or used anything they knew about me to try to ruin my life.

Safe, Sane, and Consensual (SSC): This is the basic 'law of the land' by which we tend to govern ourselves. Those engaging in play or a D/s relationship need to do so in a safe manner, with sane persons (defined as having unimpaired clarity of thought and the ability to make sound judgments), and consent to negotiated activities.

Risk-Aware Consensual Kink (RACK): This is for the more extreme 'edge-play' relationships or scenes. Those who practice RACK take things to the next level and many may find these activities beyond their limits, uncomfortable to participate in, or to even watch at times. It's important to realize that those who are engaged in such scenes or relationships still need to do so consensually and are completely aware that their actions or the situations they encounter can be risky or dangerous. This is not the type of play a novice (on either side of the coin) should plunge into and is typically restricted to those with extensive knowledge about the scenes they perform.

Consensual Non-Con (Con/NonCon): The lifestyle's biggest oxymoron and a topic of great debate is whether a person should always have the ability to say "no." A non-con (non-consensual) scene infringes upon the basic rules the lifestyle community established for safety. The risk of something going terribly wrong without the ability to realize the person truly needs to stop the scene, or that nothing is done without consent (even if consent was given previously) can still be wrong. Others argue consenting to engage in something that could be construed as non-consenting later (such as rape, kidnapping, or interrogation scenes) is still, by default, consenting to the act and therefore truly isn't a non-con act. Whichever end of the debate you may personally find yourself, this is a term that is used. When someone references being interested in Con Non-Con they typically mean an interest in activities such as arranging a kidnapping and rape-type of scene. Something where the submissive and dominant discuss, arrange, and agree to a variety of things ahead of time except for when it will happen and, once it does happen, there is no calling it off. Some feel that any element of being allowed to end/call off the activities whether it's a Safe Word, gesture, or some other means removes the non-con element and it's just a really intense staged scene. Again, this is not something people should engage in lightly especially with any of those involved being new to the scene, and it's strongly recommended that the dominant and submissive both speak to others who have done similar scenes and kinds of activities.

Safe Word: It is important to have a safe word in place *before* playing, whether for just one scene or a long-term D/s dynamic. This is a word the submissive and dominant have agreed will immediately stop any activity and end the scene completely. In most cases **Red** means "stop immediately, something is wrong, or I'm at my maximum point." **Yellow** means "slow it down I'm reaching my breaking point." **Green** is "everything feels wonderful keep going." These are common words and somewhat universal. They're good to use if you're at a play party or engaging with someone you haven't played with before. Often they're used straight up, alone and by themselves so the intention is clear. In some instances, players won't use words to indicate green/yellow (all's well/slow down) for any number of reasons. However, they still have the emergency "end everything" word but pick one that would truly stand out during a scene such as "elephant" or "asparagus" or "Mississippi."

Safety Signal: This is just like the Safe Word but for those instances when the submissive is unable to speak such as using gags or has the potential to go so into sub space that they cannot speak. Options include giving the submissive something (like a bandana) to hold in their hand and if they release it that's the stop signal. Yes, there's a chance it may be dropped in error but the dominant's job is to immediately stop and check on the submissive. If they say they dropped it in error and want to keep going then the dominant can easily put the item back in the submissive's hand and keep going. A dominant should **never** assume the item was dropped in error and ignore it.

Sub-space: This is, simply, the euphoria one reaches when they let go during a scene. Some have reported it as a sense of flying. The endorphins have kicked in and the submissive is, essentially, riding a natural high. See "headspace" for submissives.

It's important to make sure that the dominant knows what they're doing and can read the submissive's body language. In sub space, it's very easy for a submissive to no longer feel things the way they normally would and that includes pain and other warnings from their body that something is wrong. A dominant who is in-tune with their submissive (or play partner) should be able to understand the body language and get a sense for if things are not right and stop the scene on their own. Alternatively, you don't want a dominant who's so new and nervous that at the slightest whimper or flinch they stop the scene needlessly.

Aftercare: While many dominants provide aftercare, some do not, and this could be a major deciding factor for you. Aftercare is the attention a dominant gives a submissive after a scene, whether cuddling, providing drinks, something to eat (many find they need sugar-based foods), or just a safe warm place in which to "come down" out of "sub space." Scenes can be extremely intense emotionally as well as physically and some submissives feel that aftercare is an absolute must, so it's important for you to know how your would-be dominant feels about this since it's not always a given.

Sub-drop: This is often not touched upon with beginners and has been known to take many by surprise. After a scene, either minutes or even days later, a submissive can have a sudden "drop" of endorphins and experience a "crash" of sorts. This manifests as moodiness, a sudden sense of vulnerability, a need to snuggle or cuddle a lot, or even an outbreak of sudden tears. Men and women can experience sub-drop although they might do so in slightly different ways. Either way, if a sudden mood change or something "not quite the usual" happens within a few days of intense scenes it should be monitored and it's important that a submissive inform their dominant.

Hurt vs. Harm: It's important to understand that these are two different things within the lifestyle. In most cases, the term 'hurt' is seen as a good thing. It's often denoted to mean the feelings derived from a scene and the oxymoron expression "hurts so good" is alive and well in our lifestyle. Harm, however, is the one to watch out for and avoid. To harm someone could mean that they were hurt beyond their tolerance, that a safe word was ignored, or that they were in some other way put in a situation or made to experience something that was outside the realm with which they are comfortable or to which they consented. While the word 'hurt' can also be used to indicate something negative you may come across those who say things like, "I will hurt you, but I will not harm you."

YMMV: While you could encounter this in a variety of ways you will likely come across this in message forums or at discussion-based/educational-type events. It simply means Your Mileage May Vary. Everyone is different, uses tools differently, engages in their dynamic differently, and outcomes can change depending on a variety of factors. It's also sometimes used as a bit of a disclaimer. When someone is talking about how to do something or how they've done/experienced something they may put the YMMV disclaimer just to denote that what they're saying pertains to them and someone else may have a very different opinion or experience.

YKINMK: Your Kink Is Not My Kink can be seen as-is or with the addition of "ATOK" (And That's Okay) or "BTOK" (But That's Okay). If you're talking to people you may see this pop up as a way to politely say they're not into whatever you're into but they aren't judging you for it. Unfortunately, there are still people who judge others in a lifestyle that's meant to be about expressing yourself in ways that typical society would judge negatively. Judgment is the last thing we need more of so some people will throw this acronym out to let others know that while they may not have the same interests, it's a pretty judgment-free zone as long as it's respected in turn to not push your kink on others or judge them for not being interested in what you enjoy.

NSA: This stands for No Strings Attached and is a straight-to-the-point declaration that they are not looking for a relationship or anything serious. It's often a one-time hook-up situation for sex or scening but it doesn't also have to be one-time only. It could be someone looking for several get-togethers with people as long as it's understood that there is no relationship involved. They engage with someone for the sex or scene (or both), enjoy some company, and then everyone goes about their separate ways with no expectations of keeping in touch unless it's to arrange another hook-up.

Acronyms have always been popular in the lifestyle and there's a certain level of kink-specific terminology and no one is expecting you to know them all instantly. In fact, acronyms are being created and used constantly so if you don't know what something means just ask and someone will be happy to let you know the meaning.

Chapter 4

What Is A Dominant?

Perhaps one of the most frequent causes of conflict that dominants face when submissives contact us is due to the fact that the submissives seem to have the wrong image of dominants in their head. Pornography has been around almost since the beginning of human-time, and it didn't take long for the iconic image of a leather-clad, high-heeled, whip-wielding dominatrix to be born. It is an image that in this lifestyle many repeatedly try to dispel. There are other images that are equated with the lifestyle such as the big bear leather daddy although this doesn't seem to have as much of a negative impact nor is it assumed that every male dominant is expected to look or behave that way.

In many cases, a submissive (normally males) has a specific image of what a dominant (typically FemDoms) is and that idea is perpetuated by what they see when web searching for almost anything BDSM related. A submissive who seeks a female dominant may find their searches online inundated with images of a statuesque woman, slender, with breasts that are large and perky (almost disproportionately so), wearing a corset and leather boots with astronomically high heels while carrying an implement of pain such as a crop or whip and assume that's what everyone looks and behaves like. Ironically, there are also a great many images of FemDoms in collars and even more strangely out of character sometimes in posture collars, which are very rigid and uncomfortable and not at all what a dominant would wear. The Internet image of a dominatrix portrays her as strict, harsh, mean, cruel, and unrelenting. The illusion is that these women are so superior that to even have a conversation with a male is beneath them and that only orders and words of humiliation would ever be spoken to a male.

Alternatively, a submissive seeking a male dominant may find a well-muscled man bare-chested with a leather vest and pants also holding some kind of tool of the trade. He is often displayed with a woman in supplication before him. Throw in a cigar and bear-like qualities and you have a fairly common gay dominant image.

Again, in most cases, the male dominant stereotypes aren't as damaging as the FemDom image. It should be of no great surprise that men are often given greater acceptance to look however they want and to break out of the porn-molds whereas should a FemDom not look like what porn has depicted it can shatter many submissives' fantasies. These exaggerated images of dominants do exist and dominants enjoy embracing the more iconic looks, but it should never be expected that a dominant should look or act in any specific way just because that's what you saw in some kinky porn.

So what **does** a dominant look like? Well, they could be short, tall, average, thin, fat, nicely figured, black hair, red hair, and... well, I'm sure you get the point. They look just like everyone else and come in all shapes, sizes, and races. It's important to realize that while a dominant can and does possess whips, crops, corsets, vests, leather boots, or any other parts of the pre-conceived image, it is not the attire or accouterments that make them a dominant. In fact, dominants often have different styles for different kinds of events ranging from everyday attire to small gatherings to full-blown fetish events.

One of the most important things a submissive should understand is that the *appearance* of being dominant doesn't mean they really are a dominant. I've found an alarming amount of profiles for submissives that specifically state in order to be "dominant enough" for them to consider the dominant they must have a certain number of toys/tools. Purchasing a slew of tools/toys just means they have money to spend and little else. Just because someone can buy the outfit and associated accouterments that take only a click of a button or a swipe of the credit card doesn't mean they know anything about using them, how to do so safely, or how to dominate in general. Some of the most amazing dominants I've known could create entire scenes from just a few things from a dollar store. Others have been able to make a submissive reach some of the most intense sub space with no costumes and just their voice and hands. Let's all remember that a big bank account and a fully stocked dungeon is not a prerequisite for being a dominant, unlike what a certain set of books/movies (that are actually rather shunned by the community in general) may trick you into thinking otherwise.

The biggest thing a submissive needs to remember is that a dominant is a person just like everyone else. They can look like anyone you see on the streets or they could be someone you interact with every day and never even realize who they are at home. In fact, many of them hold average jobs whether working in an office, as a CEO of a company, as the cleaning lady, or as a store clerk. Yes, it's true; some wonderful dominants hold jobs that are certainly less-than-glamorous or can even be some way non-dominating. Not every dominant is the top executive at their company and might be your neighbor barista. Some are mothers and fathers who work the lifestyle around raising children. Some are married and are successful at integrating D/s into their marriages and lives in general. I've known many in long-term relationships or marriages who take on a submissive for one or for both partners and many who manage to incorporate a successful poly dynamic, albeit this is a difficult dynamic to maintain.

Not every dominant is straight and, in fact, many in the lifestyle have a very fluid outlook on sexuality. There are butches and lesbians who may be seeking male submissives. Just because a woman identifies as butch doesn't necessarily mean she's a lesbian, she may well be, but there are certainly plenty of straight butches out there who love their male submissives dearly. A seemingly straight male who only takes on female submissives may not be averse to playing with a male even in a sensual way. Remember that gender and sexuality are all on spectrums and add incredible diversity to a wonderful community. I know, I know, all the blurring of terms and lines can make a person's head spin. All the more reason to not head into your search with too many physical ideals as it will be very difficult to find the exact image you've conjured.

The best rule of thumb is - Never Assume. Don't assume they are a sadist, straight, gay, or what title they prefer. The vital part here is to make sure you do your own due diligence before you make your first approach. Remember, most people will appreciate you inquiring how they prefer to be addressed rather than you willy-nilly calling all FemDoms mistress or all male dominants master. There have been more than enough instances when a male has addressed all women as mistress including submissive women, and while most will correct you it does show that you're not interested in learning about anyone, and in particular, you're just hoping to shoot into the dark and hopefully win yourself a mistress. It usually tells everyone you just emailed: all you did was copy/paste a message and sent it to anyone who had female or dominant in their profile instead of actually reading each profile. Remember, this is a life-goal, not a carnival.

When you contact a dominant it's important to realize that at the other end there is not a dominant sitting upon a throne decked out in leather with dutiful servants bustling about doing their bidding. Chances are you are emailing someone who just got home from work, has to cook dinner, put the kids to bed, make lunch for tomorrow, and do the laundry before throwing themselves exhaustedly into bed just to do it all over again in the morning. If you're looking for that leather-clad god/dess seek out a professional dominant and they'll be more than happy to put on whatever outfit your mind can conjure up... for the right price. If you're looking for someone for a more long-term dynamic and deeper connection then remember you're speaking to a real person who has their own needs and desires and is seeking someone who fits their own wants.

Dominants come in all shapes, sizes, work backgrounds, and financial statuses. What they are **not** is that pornographic image you see splattered all over the Internet. Once you get yourself more firmly grounded in reality the more genuine your interactions will become and the better your odds become at making the connection you truly seek and, at the very least, making some new and fun friends along the way.

Chapter 5

Female-Led Relationships in A Male-Led Society

Originally I included a chapter on this subject for the male submissive seeking female dominant version of the book, but I've opted to include it (with appropriate revisions) in this version as much has come to light in our society in the last couple of years and I feel this still is important to include.

Our society puts a lot of expectations on gender despite being narrowly focused on just the gender binary (cis male and cis female) and how those "two genders" are to look and behave. In the last couple of years, in particular, there have been great strides to *Break the Binary* and educate the world that gender is a spectrum and fluid. I will go into further detail about this in the next chapter, so this chapter is more focused on how societal norms are no longer the status quo and how our community needs to not just be aware of that but embrace it without necessarily giving up our own individual desires.

Despite the tremendous amount of publicity made toward the gender equality movement (most often specifically albeit a little limited in its focus on acknowledging, treating, and paying women as equals to men) there's far too much inequality still ahead of us. It is, unfortunately, still assumed that being a woman automatically is equated with being weaker, less-than, and submissive to men. Although this lifestyle is very much about exploring yourself, being whomever (or whatever) you want to be, and no judgment and often reveres women, there are still far too many who maintain this "women = less" mentality. We see this in the fetish of *forced feminization.*

One good thing about the lifestyle is that women are equally dominants and have a subset of the D/s lifestyle dedicated to them as such. Female-Led Relationships (FLR) are incredibly popular and common in the lifestyle and this has been so for countless years. It's important for submissive men in this dynamic to understand that women are often not considered or treated as equals in society overall, and a good way to honor women is to help promote more gender equality for women.

In most cases, this mentality has been so thoroughly ingrained into the mindset of society that people do not even realize they do or say things that indicate that the female is 'secondary.' Perhaps one of the easiest real-life examples would be while dining out. While most wait-staff don't give it a second thought or even "mean anything by it" they will often defer to the male, especially when presenting the check or asking if the table needs anything. A good way to navigate a situation like this is for you, the submissive male, to defer immediately to the female dominant and often it takes only a look to the dominant for the wait-staff to take the hint.

The next few times that you're out with any female in your life observe the wait-staff carefully. Not always, but most commonly, they will approach and direct their body in some way towards the male while asking if everything is okay or to whom the check should be given. Once the look is given to the dominant, or female in general, you can usually see the wait-staff adjust their body to acknowledge her preferential status.

Geography can play a part in how others perceive a female and a male together. In New York and similar metropolitan areas they're often regarded equally or even with the female being deferred to, while in the South, people are more apt to address males first. Explore your own area and see where the sensor for this falls and use opportunities while you're out with friends to gauge (and even correct) this type of behavior.

Women have come a long way in recent years, taking on positions of authority that were previously exclusive to men. Society as a whole is becoming more aware and accepting of the power of women but there are still people in some areas of the country (and government) for whom the male is the dominant figure and that's just "how it should be." When dealing with attitudes such as these there can rarely be an understanding of kink and D/s dynamics, and some people (especially other men) will perceive a submissive male to be not even a man. It could be cause for social ridicule or even physical challenge to the male submissive.

While this isn't a dissertation on society, it's hard not to apply some of those same principles when we're forced to deal with the outside vanilla world. It's important for a male submissive to realize that certain areas or groups may find behavior that acknowledges a woman or allows the woman to call the shots extremely emasculating and they will make that fact known… often loudly and obnoxiously. This could be exciting for someone who truly enjoys emasculation and humiliation, but overall it's childish posturing on the other person's part and could lead to unwanted attention or even physical altercations.

Not everyone will make an issue of a man deferring to a woman and most people are far too absorbed in their own lives to even notice. However, the fact remains that women do still struggle in a "man's world" no matter how subtle or overt that conflict may be.

In this chapter I want you, the male submissive, to not just read and acknowledge that this does happen but to try some of these real-world experiments.

1. Take a female friend out to eat a few times. Each time closely observe the body language and positioning of the wait-staff when speaking to either of you. Jot down some of your observations to remember later.

2. Accompany a female friend to such male-oriented businesses as a mechanic, car dealership, or hardware store. Note how the sales people or mechanics direct the discussion toward you, the male. Try it a few times at different types of establishments and experiment. Try standing beside her, try standing behind her, try looking attentive, and try looking distracted. How frequently are you still addressed preferentially over your female friend?

3. While this may be more of a geographical issue, listen closely to how women are spoken to at a male-oriented location (as in #2). Do men speaking to her address her politely as Miss or Ma'am or does she get the "little lady" treatment?

4. As you encounter instances when you are automatically deferred to, try a little exercise by learning to defer the conversation to your

female friend. Unless she is specifically looking for your assistance in negotiations or understanding (such as in an area you are specifically skilled), try to bring the attention of the sales staff back to your friend.

Despite there being some places where the male rules the roost, many may applaud your deferring to the female as an act of chivalry. In fact, chivalry should be an important goal and frequent tool in your daily life, which will go a long way to enhancing your D/s dynamic once you establish one. Not only are you being a gentleman, but you are also providing a service.

Chapter 6

TGNC – Not A Fetish

First, let's explain what TGNC stands for and what it means. While many have begun to hear about transgender, many don't realize being transgender is just one aspect of the gender spectrum. As with sexuality being far more than just gay, straight, lesbian, or bisexual gender is equally vast and complex. Discussion about the gender and sexuality spectrums (and they are two separate things) can easily fill books on their own so this will be just a quick crash course to help you avoid some pitfalls and perhaps be a foundation for you to explore additional resources to learn more and become a better person and an ally.

The first thing you may realize is that I typically keep using TGNC instead of just transgender and that's because TGNC is a more inclusive umbrella term which stands for Transgender Gender Non-Conforming. Being transgender is just one possible way in which a person can gender identify, and while transgender people have received an incredible amount of publicity in the last couple of years due to a show-off (who does not represent the trans community and therein will be unnamed) and thanks to others who had a positive influence like Laverne Cox, Chaz Bono, Carmen Carrera, Lily and Lana Wachowski and countless other brave souls who brought positive attention about being transgender to the general population, trans people aren't the only ones out there. In fact, we can now see others within the TGNC community being seen in media with such names as Asia Kate Dillon (non-binary) from shows like *Orange is the New Black* and *Billions*, Ezra Miller (queer, gender fluid) who is perhaps most notably known as Barry Allen/The Flash in the DC movies, specifically *Justice League*. Rose McGowan (non-binary) who was popularly known for her role on *Charmed* or in Tarantino's *Grindhouse* movies. There is also the incomparable Tilda Swinton (gender fluid) who has a substantial repertoire but may be more currently best known for being the White Witch in the *Chronicles of Narnia* films or the Ancient One in *Doctor Strange*.

While I won't list the myriad ways in which someone can gender identify because there are, in fact, so many and even new ones being introduced at times, I will strongly advise you to look deeper into this subject. The best advice I can give to you is to never assume someone's gender, never question the way in which they wish to express that gender, and never assume someone's pronouns. A TGNC person will always appreciate you asking "what pronouns do you use" over just assuming and using the wrong ones. Remember, it's not a binary world anymore so he/him and she/her pronouns aren't the only pronouns available anymore.

The terminology around the TGNC community can seem daunting but it should be something everyone strives to at least look into and respect. One area that seems to be confusing but is actually pretty straightforward is that gender and sexuality are completely different things.

Special note: If you are a TGNC person who may be triggered by some of the derogatory words that were/are associated with the TGNC community avoid page 43 as I have included them as a warning of what NOT to say to a TGNC person.

Terminology

Transgender/Trans: Someone who was assigned a gender at birth but feels this is wrong and identifies as the opposite gender.

Trans woman/Trans female/MtF: A person who was assigned male at birth but identifies as a woman.

Trans man/Trans male/FtM: A person who was assigned female at birth but identifies as a man.

Intersex: A person who is born with more than one gender-type sex characteristic internally and/or externally.

Cisgender/Cis man/Cis female: A person who feels in alignment with and identifies as the gender in which they were assigned at birth.

(Gender) Dysphoria: What many (albeit not all) non-cisgender people feel. It can manifest in different ways for different people to different degrees of severity, but it's generally the emotional turmoil associated with being in the "wrong body."

The Surgery: There is no singular surgery. There is no such thing as "the surgery." Trans women and trans men have the option to have a variety of surgical procedures to help them feel more in alignment with their body.

Gender Affirming Surgery: This is the more accurate term. It was previously known as Gender Reassignment Surgery (GRS) or Sex Reassignment Surgery (SRS) but that has since been changed to Gender Affirming Surgery. This could be one or multiple procedures that go toward helping a trans person feel more in line with the gender in which they identify.

TGNC: Transgender/Gender Non-Conforming is the umbrella term in which to identify anyone who is not cisgender.

Gender Binary: Binary is the 0s and 1s which are the absolute foundation that makes up everything digital and has been used to illustrate that society assumes there are only two genders – (cis) male and female. This is not the case in reality and therein you may encounter *Break the Binary* and similar terms which are intended to point out that gender is a spectrum.

There are countless ways in which a person can identify their gender other than cis male/cis female or trans male/transfemale. There's gender queer, gender fluid, agender, two-spirit (which is just for native/indigenous people), bigender, androgynous and the list goes on.

Regardless of how someone identifies, it's their body and life and therefore is only for them to determine. Do not try to "correct" someone about their gender identity or tell them that they don't look close enough to their gender identity (i.e. passing or not passable).

A TGNC person could discover they're not cisgender at an incredibly young age like one well-known trans advocate, while others have gone their entire lives only to more recently discover it (or be brave enough to express it) as we saw in *Transparent* (2014 - 2019). Given the stigma attached to being anything other than a straight cisgender person in previous decades many had to hide their true selves for many different reasons and were only able to come out later in life. Additionally, it's important to realize that a person does not have to undergo surgical procedures or hormone replacement therapy to be "considered" transgender because there is no one way (or right way) to be any gender or in how to express one's gender.

What TGNC people are **not**, however, is a fetish. The porn industry has done significant damage to the TGNC community by making and promoting content that makes being a TGNC person into a fetish and often by using derogatory terms (discussed below). The people used in the videos are real TGNC people who may feel that this is one of the few businesses in which they can be themselves without being completely alienated and this was (and still is) a very real concern for TGNC people. In most places in the United States and other countries, you can still be fired for being other than heterosexual so it's not surprising that there are a vast number of places and companies that do not protect their TGNC employees. Further, the TGNC community is one of the most likely to be homeless and many have been forced into some kind of sex work in order to survive. This isn't an issue that's a few decades old and has since been corrected, this is a very real issue that many TGNC, especially the youth demographic, face today. As such, sex work and porn content have become a way in which to get any kind of work. They are forced not only to sell themselves but to sell their dignity as they are often subjected to being the "bottom" or "used/abused" or otherwise subservient type in the porn content because they're not a cisgender person.

There are some amazing adult performers who are in the TGNC community who have made it a point to perform in and produce sex-positive adult content. They do not engage in this content because they're forced and therein have no control over how they're represented. Instead, they have embraced their bodies, their gender, and their sexualities to create consenting adult content that promotes positive content. Buck Angel is among the most famous of the TGNC adult performers and has dedicated his life to being a positive influence on sex, sexuality, and gender and has done a lot to educate across the world.

I want to take a moment to explain that some TGNC people actually do like to be fetishized and will actively seek this out. Some are also interested in being humiliated and degraded because they are TGNC (similar to race-play). It's vital that everyone understand that, as with most things in life, there's always the exception to the rule and this is the case here. While it's not unheard of it is extremely rare to encounter a TGNC person who seeks out this type of interaction. As such, it's always best to assume the TGNC person does **not** want to be a fetish or degraded for being TGNC and should always be treated like every other person. While this book is geared towards those who are submissive and are seeking a dominant, it's not unheard of for TGNC dominants to be fetishized and it seems that trans women get a significant amount of this fetishization.

Along these lines, it's also important to point out that TGNC people and those interested in forced feminization/sissification or cross-dressing are completely different. Some of this has been addressed in other chapters but it's important to emphasize that feminization/sissification and cross-dressing are fetishes while being TGNC is the way in which a human being identifies.

It's also very important to be aware that trans people can be very dysphoric about their genitals so pay close attention to the way in which they refer to themselves and those parts. Not mentioning genitals can also be just as telling. While there are plenty of trans guys who love penetration in either hole, many trans men do not want to even acknowledge their "front hole" and have no desire to be penetrated there and might only enjoy anal sex or not enjoy penetration of any kind. Trans women may often reference their genitals as clits or their anus as a vagina. Do not ask about how a TGNC person refers to their genitals in the first couple of emails and let some trust build before even thinking of broaching this subject and when you do, make sure you proceed with extreme caution and the utmost respect. Don't ask things like "What will I be sucking," or "What do you call your holes," but rather try some respect and tact with something like: "I don't want to cause you any dysphoria, but whenever you feel comfortable could you please tell me how you wish to have certain things referred to so I don't misspeak or offend you?"

Avoid prefacing questions with: "I don't mean to be rude but…" because odds are if you have to make such a disclaimer you are, in fact, being rude. Remember, a lot of information can be found online and you really should access those resources before asking a TGNC person questions that might be invasive. Hearing: "I looked up some more information online and I was a little confused about x, y, z and would love to learn more if you feel comfortable talking about it," is a million times better than prefacing rude questions.

<u>Derogatory Terms</u>

Here's a brief list of words that you **<u>should not</u>** use when speaking to or about anyone who is or may be TGNC. Even if you hear/see someone else use any of these do not think this gives you license to do it as well. Even if the TGNC person uses any of these terms this is not permission for you to use them either.

- Tranny

- Transvestite/Transvestism

- She-male/He-she/Shim/She-it

- That/Thing/It

Other words that are wrong or that should be avoided include:

- Transgendered/Transgenderism – there are no such things. It would be the same thing as calling someone heterosexualed.

- Sex change – This is no longer appropriate and has another term (as mentioned above). However, it's typically not acceptable to discuss someone's genitals and what surgical procedures they had/will have.

- Biological/genetic – Phrasing something as "biological" or "genetic" gender is antiquated and inappropriate. It's more properly phrased as "gender assigned at birth."

- Trap – this is used when an (ignorant) person feels they were "duped" or "trapped" by a TGNC person once they find out the person was assigned another gender at birth because the person was so "passable." This implies that the TGNC person is pretending or deceiving someone about their own gender rather than acknowledging it for being the bigoted statement that it is.

- Reverse Genital Terms: Do not call a trans man's chest "breasts/tits" or his bottom part "vagina/pussy." Do not call a trans woman's bottom parts "cock/penis" and so forth. As the lifestyle is meant to be intimate and often is highly sexual you can ask the TGNC person what words they prefer for different parts. Once they tell you, that's it – end of discussion. Do not use other terms because you think it's more fitting.

General Things to Avoid Saying

While you may think it's a compliment, do not bring up how well a TGNC person "passes" because you are calling attention to the fact that you see them as other than the gender in which they identify or that they have to look a certain way in order to be considered that gender. Do not ask a TGNC person how they will be having sex with you or how you will have sex with them. Aside from it being a rude and ignorant question, it's also something anyone with common sense could figure out. Do not ask them what bathroom they use. Do not assume that a trans man likes to be penetrated. Many trans men do love to be penetrated, others prefer only anal penetration, while others prefer no penetration at all.

Typically I'm a proponent of "When in doubt – ask," but the way people ask and certain things that get asked can be really troublesome to some TGNC people. If you're curious about something it's probably better to look it up online first and that means using legitimate resources and not porn-based sites. If you're still trying to learn further a good way to approach the subject would be:

Sir/Ma'am, I've tried looking up a few resources but I'm not sure if this is accurate or if it's what you think/feel. I have a couple of questions that I would like to ask only so that I can be better informed and grow as a person.

While the TGNC community is incredibly vast and complex, it's very important that everyone (regardless of where you stand in the lifestyle or life in general) do a little research in order to learn and be more sensitive to trans people and what not to say. Be an ally! There are more TGNC people than you think and there very well may be someone in your own life who is TGNC (whether they're out or not).

Bottom-line – the TGNC people are not here to be your fetishes. They are not here to be demeaned, degraded, humiliated, or in any other way physically or verbally abused.

Chapter 7

WATCH OUT!
Bad or Fake Dominants

Chances are you're focusing your search almost entirely online at this point. If so, you've undoubtedly come across a few websites that specifically cater to the lifestyle at-large and probably a few others that cater to specific areas of interest (fetish-specific). If you haven't yet, odds are you will encounter a vast array of fakes, scam artists, and cyber players soon enough. The ruses are often fairly transparent but sometimes can be rather elaborate and difficult to detect. Unfortunately, only time and experience will help you weed out the fakes, but in the interim here are some tips to help you avoid some common pitfalls.

Pictures: It is extraordinarily easy for anyone to snatch an image from the web and post it to a profile. There are some websites and browser add-on's to assist in discovering if a photograph has been posted elsewhere by doing reverse image searches. If a photo seems professionally captured or too good to be true then chances are… it is. Many professional models or even non-models who happen to be rather good-looking whether they be male or female or whether they do fetish work or not have their pictures stolen and used to create fake profiles. I found one where the woman's picture was from a hunting show that had her image taken and used on a kink site for a profile. It was immediately removed when I reported the theft to the original owner thanks to reverse image searches. Check the image to see if it's been uploaded somewhere else and look for photo-tampering or similar evidence. More on how to use tools and searches below.

Fakes: Not necessarily to be confused with the scam artists, although fake profiles can often involve scams. Fake profiles are generally created by men and usually feature images of gorgeous women, typically between the ages of 18 and 25 who reside in major U.S. cities like Miami, San Francisco, and New York City. Many times they will lure people in for nothing more than a quick cyber jerk-off session but sometimes they do it to gain gifts and money. At least one male has come forward openly in forums bragging about how he rarely has to pay for anything because of his scam based on an entirely fake female profile.

Scams: This includes paying for sessions (either online or in person) whether they promote themselves as a professional dominant or not. It often results in the scammer never showing up or disappearing (ghosting) altogether. Some scams have been known to go so far as to have the submissive take out lines of credit for the "Mistress" to use at-will, while the submissive waits for a never-to-happen encounter. Some come through with a few teaser cyber sessions, especially if they think the 'mark' can and will give them more or bigger things.

Many times you're dealing with a male and usually someone with little to no real interest or experience in the lifestyle beyond what they've read about online. Phone calls or webcam sessions can be staged enlisting the help of a female friend in exchange for a cut of the loot. This is especially true if the "Mistress" doesn't allow you to call her except at very specific dates and times or they insist on calling you. When they do call you their number comes up as blocked, private, or restricted giving you no ability to contact the person in return. This allows the scam-artist time to arrange a female to act the part for voice or "cam" verification and doesn't allow many options for the duped submissive to track them down.

This can happen to female submissives although it's much less likely. Women are already inherently more cautious due to the constant risks they face just because they're female and most understand that identifying as a submissive makes them an even greater target. Having to develop a savvy and cautionary mentality because of how society is in general already helps them avoid scams like this in many cases. So, while scammers can and do target females, it's just less likely to occur or go too far before the female catches on to the scam.

This doesn't mean you should never ever give gifts to your dominant, but it does mean you should exercise caution. If you're seeing a professional dominant with a reliable reputation and you establish a history of satisfying engagements then feel free to throw in an extra gift whenever possible. Even a little trinket to a dominant you've met a few times and are hoping to see again is a nice gesture. But never, ever, ever offer your credit (lines of credit, credit cards, signing your name to a loan) to someone with whom you don't have a long, trusted, and well-established relationship.

<u>Fake Pro-Dominants</u>: Anyone who is a genuine professional has considerable skill, experience, safety protocols, and an even/calm temperament. Someone who doesn't have these qualities is likely someone looking to make a quick buck and that's what makes them not just a fake but also dangerous.

What makes a fake pro-dominant a bit different from a scammer is that they are actually willing to perform domination in exchange for the money or gifts given, however, they may not know anything about what they're doing. This is a good way for someone to get hurt... badly. A wayward crack of a single-tail whip can easily cause serious physical damage. Tying someone up isn't just a matter of wrapping a lot of rope around them, it's a matter of paying very close attention to the submissive to ensure that there are no circulation issues, observing, being aware, and stopping if the submissive hits their limits that even they may not be cognizant of reaching (typically due to subspace and not realizing what's going on with their body).

A fake will be happy to crack a whip, dress the part, stomp on you, or whatever else you ask for, in exchange for your cash, and you **may** get lucky enough to not get hurt in a non-kinky way but you are taking a good risk here. A "new" professional dominant will likely 'apprentice' under an experienced professional before going solo. Thanks to the endless resources online anyone can watch videos and read websites to learn the basics and there is a good deal that's common sense (i.e. paddling or spanking someone), but what far too many how-to videos fail to cover are safety aspects including where you should and should not strike or what to do if something goes wrong. As such, those who just feel this is a quick and fun way to make under the table cash and gifts will fall into this category. Not only should they be avoided because of their lack of skills but also because they typically have no real interest in the lifestyle and therein are not looking to establish an actual D/s relationship.

FinDominants (Financial Domination): As previously mentioned, this is different than a pro-dominant in that their entire goal is to seek money and gifts with little to no effort expended on their part. The most common prey of a FinDominant is someone who enjoys humiliation, as a FinDominant needs only to mock them or tell them to do things with little actual input or much action on their part and then they can sit back and reap their rewards. The plague of FinDominants on certain websites has made many submissives extremely hesitant in future dealings, and rightly so. Some FinDominants will even refuse to speak to a would-be submissive without some type of money or tribute "for their precious time" spent simply exchanging emails. While they may fill a need for a select few, overall this is a large scam and, again, usually run by men pretending to be women, or just really lazy people looking for a quick cash payout.

Not only is this very common among male submissives seeking female dominants but it's especially common among gay men, although there are plenty of times either the "top" and/or the "submissive" identify as straight. There are countless sites and profiles dedicated to brutish men happy to humiliate submissive men in exchange for cash or gifts. This is also common around specific fetishes like socks, jock straps, and other popular gay interests. In some cases, the submissive doesn't necessarily identify as a gay man and will, in fact, identify as a straight man who feels that being treated harshly or humiliated by another man extremely emasculating and that is exactly what they seek.

Regardless of sexuality or gender this is unfortunately a very common practice by people who figured out there are people who are either ill-equipped with Internet safety practices or are just so desperate to get their own kinks met that they just don't care about who is really on the other end of the chat and they are willing to pay up for any attention. If both parties are aware that this is strictly a financial arrangement such as a person wanting to just be tormented online for a bit, pay up, and then disconnect with no complications then that's something both parties consent to and is perfectly fine. However, it's when people are using the guise of being a dominant but only for money and have no intention of actually being a dominant or in other ways deceive the unsuspecting submissive is where this practice is wrong and should be avoided at all costs.

A Word About References

If someone states they have references (or even that they currently have a submissive in their service) and then follows up with something along the lines of, "but you can't talk them," this is a clear indication that something is wrong. Anyone worthwhile, professional or lifestyler alike, will let you contact their references if they have any to offer. Just because a person doesn't have references doesn't mean they aren't legit or won't be a wonderful dominant, it's the person who makes a claim that they have references but then tries to hide them that should be an immediate red flag.

Additionally, the dominant will allow you to contact these references at random and without them being present so you or the references won't feel intimidated. Allowing you to contact them at random means there's a greater likelihood that the dominant isn't posing as these other people just to give favorable reviews. They may also invite you to openly attend various events or groups they attend so you can watch how they engage with people, how others engage with them, and give you the opportunity to speak to references in a more personal setting.

Since references are provided by other people in the lifestyle, a degree of privacy and discretion is well advised however willing they are to vouch for the dominant. This may mean that all you get is an email address or username and website for the reference person as they are entitled to their own privacy. This is not an immediate "red flag" that you have encountered a scam, but a means to ensure the privacy of those you contact. This means emails through BDSM sites versus getting any private addresses or phone numbers might be what you get since inputting a person's email address can yield access to someone's information online. Once you explain that you'd like to discuss the perspective dominant or professional you are considering, the references may opt to provide you with more personal methods of contact. Remember, while you and the dominant have been conversing these people don't know you at all and should not be expected to release their private information.

If phone numbers or personal emails are included guard this information with your life and, in fact, dispose of it properly after you're satisfied. Seeing phone numbers makes it easier to quell your fears and know you're speaking to a real person who is not the dominant/professional posing under alternate emails. Once more, I cannot emphasize enough that just because you don't get someone's phone number for reference purposes doesn't necessarily mean there's a conspiracy to dupe you.

General Safety

It is also a good idea to ask if the dominant/professional is a member of local groups. Attending or arranging the first meet at such a gathering/munch, gives you a better chance of getting legitimate references. If the dominant/professional offers to have you attend a function to have a more intimate interaction and/or play, this is a wonderful opportunity but remember you do not have to get intimate or do any scenes that you're uncomfortable with and, in fact, this should be avoided on your first meet-up.

Hearing things like, "I'm shy so I don't talk to that many people in real life," is a cue that something is not right. If they are a dominant chances are they are not *that* shy. That's not to say dominants can't be shy (as I've known a few who can be painfully shy), but typically they have the ability to interact with people in general and are willing to attend events, munches, or at the very least have a private group of select friends in the lifestyle you can contact.

If someone is completely without a reference it shouldn't be a deal breaker but you should definitely be leery. "I just moved here so there's no one for you to call," is another warning sign. It doesn't matter if they've been in town a day or a year, there should be someone at their previous location who you can get in touch with... that is, unless of course they're lying or running away from something they don't want anyone to know about.

There's a careful balance between giving someone the benefit of the doubt because things do happen in life and being skeptical. Giving a little leeway in the beginning for perhaps one or two things that could come off with a negative vibe is one thing, but if there's a pattern of evasion, inconsistent answers, and a general sense of being sneaky then it's likely better to err on the side of caution and move along. That doesn't mean you have to ghost the person or outright block them, try the upfront approach first by saying something like: "Thank you for taking the time to talk with me but I think this isn't going to pan out." If they become persistent or get nasty about it then you've gotten the chance to see their real colors and to know that you made the right call to end things at that point.

Remember, your gut is a really valuable tool and it's one that far too many people ignore. We hear countless stories where someone says: "I just had a bad feeling about it but I thought I was just being paranoid..." and in far too many instances their bad feeling/gut/instinct was right. We have an innate biological drive to stay safe and alive and that 'instinct' is not just some "New Age mumbo-jumbo" but is, instead, a critical tool we have and need to use more often. It's important to be realistic in your expectations – a dominant isn't going to give you their life story and personal contact information in the first few emails. Take a step back to see if you're pressing too hard too fast or if the way you're wording things could be considered off-putting or even too aggressive. If there's something that seems 'off' about the other person proceed with caution and use some basic common sense, but if you feel your instincts are telling you to watch out then it's always better to follow that alert.

Chapter 8

Fact vs. Fiction

There are so many stories, movies, and even TV shows/episodes that are dedicated to or have strong kink themes that it could easily take over the span of this book. There's also a great debate on what should and shouldn't be considered kink or BDSM related in popular media as there are times when BDSM is categorized as abuse while there are plenty of times that abuse is glossed over because it was said to be BDSM. Again, getting into this debate would be far beyond the scope of this book, but I wanted to touch on a few of the biggest ones that have seemed to impact the community in some way or another.

When certain books or movies are released it can cause a significant wave to ripple throughout the community. We saw this happen with the sudden popularity of the *Fifty Shades Trilogy* and the subsequent release of the films. Each time a film was about to be released the local community groups would inevitably see an influx of newbies. As with anything, some stayed, some came just once in a while, while others left a tad disappointed by the reality of the lifestyle. Bringing the lifestyle into a more mainstream audience can be a good thing as it could help the average vanilla person realize that BDSM isn't about being scared and tortured but it also gives potential newbies very unrealistic expectations. However, BDSM in media has never been portrayed well enough for the average vanilla person to accept it as being "not deviant" because it's almost always portrayed in a way that paints the people involved as criminals.

Think of how many TV shows like *Law & Order* have episodes where a victim is a "submissive" who got mixed up with an underground sex club and was tortured and either purposefully or accidentally killed. Or how many times dominants are depicted as being amoral, heartless, or even stereotypically decked out in full "dominatrix" type gear. In the episode 'The Mistress Always Spanks Twice' (S02E16) of *Castle* they played both sides of the fence a bit but predominantly showed the stereotypical images which also included only slender women and muscled men and pretty much all being white rather than the myriad of body types, races, genders – or any diversity – that's found within the lifestyle.

Gor

In 1966 John Norman introduced the world to his Gorean series which started with *Tarnsmen of Gor* and went on to include 34 books with the last one being as recent as 2016 – although there was a gap of no books throughout the 1990s. The books were developed before the moon landing so it used the premise that there was a "counter-Earth" that was hiding directly behind the moon and matched our orbit and, therein, as undetectable. Despite being Earth-like its overall design was much like most fantasy genre worlds with vast open expanses, small villages with some areas developing into cities, and men walking around with swords and animal pelts. However, some possessed the technology to travel to the real Earth wherein they would pick up people they felt would make good additions to their world, typically beautiful women (although sometimes men) who would be transported to become slaves. It is significantly geared toward "natural male dominance" mentality especially that men are entitled to be dominant over women. It does also include male slaves, female dominants, and free persons but the overall theme that runs throughout the series is male dominance.

As with many fantasy novels, John Norman crafted a world, the people, the society/caste structure, rules and laws, and terminology specific unto the world he created, with each book building upon the existing structure and expanding into greater detail. Given the significant amount of details provided on how the slaves were divided into their own hierarchy, explicit rules they had to follow, and intricate details on their behavior including specific positions and manners in which to serve, it isn't difficult to understand how this touched a chord with many interested in BDSM. Given the difficulty in finding material that could excite someone that was kink-related unless you went to pretty seedy sex shops, this series was something that anyone could get with ease and it blended in well enough with the bulk of the sci-fi/fantasy genre books being published at the time. It quickly allowed many who were interested in kink but unsure of what to do or where to start a virtual how-to guide through the myriad rules and positions described throughout the series.

Given the popularity and how long the series was running for at the time combined with the 80s being one in which sci-fi/fantasy films exploded in Hollywood, it was inevitable that the series would be picked up and made into a film. The films were created by and acted in with fairly obscure people with the exception of Jack Palance who they somehow managed to get to play Xenos, not once but twice and a quick appearance from Arnold Vosloo. *Gor* was released in February 1988 and despite incredibly poor box office sales and mostly negative reviews *Gor II* (aka *Outlaw of Gor*) somehow got made and was released in March 1989. Die-hard Gorean fans will have sought out the films but even many of them were left very unhappy with the end product. The second film got some revitalization when it was done on *Mystery Science Theater 3000* (519) in 1993 but it just illustrated how poorly done the film attempts were.

While the Internet has been around for a long time and there's been Usenet and IRC and other venues that allowed people to access venues in which to talk about kink, let's fast forward to the 1990s when AOL started to be used in households and especially around 1996-1997 when it became unlimited and allowed people, even those who never would have considered being online before, access to a whole new world. It also gave people access to chat rooms and Gor-based rooms exploded. Whether it was rooms to talk about the books, generic world of Gor, specific cities or villages in Gor, or even specific locations like taverns – they were out there and they were filled with people. For the most part, they were Role-playing Game (RPG) based rooms where users could take on a character and write out their actions and could even use specific key-entries to engage in battles. Fast forward a little more to the release of Second Life and the Gorean role-playing world takes on a whole new life of its own. If you do a search for anything Gor related online today you will find immeasurable sites dedicated to the books, the world itself, and to those who use Gor in their lifestyle.

Many folks have tried to live a Gorean lifestyle as close to the books as possible, with one group even going so far as to try to build a Gorean community on a large property. For the most part, however, those who identify as Goreans in real life are akin to those who practice a religion – it's a mindset, an overall belief system. They integrate as many aspects from the books into their lives as possible and this primarily focuses around the rules and positions of slaves (kajira/kajirus). However, those who proclaim to be Gorean within the lifestyle are often mocked or seen as not being "real" or that their kinks/lifestyles are "less," even though we shouldn't be judging others and there is no singular way to be kinky or how to live your kinky life.

Secretary/Pet

Secretary came out in 2002 and starred major actors James Spader and Maggie Gyllenhaal and performed fairly well with viewers and critics alike. On his website review of the film, Roger Ebert wrote that the movie… "approaches the tricky subject of sadomasochism with a stealthy tread, avoiding the dangers of making it either too offensive, or too funny." Additionally, he and most others lauded the performances of both actors with Spader playing Mr. Grey (yes, that's right) who is a lawyer and Gyllenhaal playing his secretary, Lee Holloway. It is often discussed and favored by those in the lifestyle as it is one of the few examples that show BDSM, especially dominance and submission, in a non-stereotypical manner nor does it indicate that sex and BDSM is the same thing. However, (and this is fairly spoiler-free) some feel that the way Mr. Grey treated Lee as we near the end was abandonment and therein abusive, but the movie is not that simple and that's one of the things that makes it still relevant.

A few years later *The Pet* was released in 2006 and created a good deal of buzz within the kink community, especially those interested in pet-play. While this was a relatively low budget film, it did have some beautiful locations and was shot fairly well and the beginning part of the story was interesting. Unfortunately, that's about where the good things for this film end. The plot had issues in general but it suddenly becomes a whole different movie partway through and immediately threw it into the typical tropes movies with BDSM use too often, which is people using the lifestyle for nefarious and non-consensual purposes. If they fleshed out a better script using the first half as the basic premise and went into more detail with the two main characters and the wife this could have been a completely different movie and would have been one of the few that didn't try to smear the lifestyle, but it failed miserably in that regard. It was also yet another depiction of wealthy people (especially those depicted as dominants) whereas the majority of the community are not ungodly rich folks.

Rich and famous people are bound to be in the lifestyle in some way or another, but media depictions seem to think only rich people can be in the lifestyle. This has never been more apparent than when *Fifty Shades* hit the shelves.

Fifty Shades Trilogy

E.L. James wrote *Twilight* fan fiction and as a result, we wound up with this trilogy that swept the world like a firestorm. When the first book was released in 2011 it was quickly followed by the next two books in 2012 and by then it wasn't just consumed by readers, it was devoured and was quickly dubbed "Mommy Porn" as the majority of the readers were women. I won't go into much detail about the overall storylines as it's become so often referenced in pop culture at this point that odds are you already know the majority of the plots. Even if you didn't read any of the books it's pretty likely that you've seen at least one trailer, if not one of the actual movies. The films *Fifty Shades of Grey, Fifty Shades Darker,* and *Fifty Shades Freed* were released right around Valentine's Day in 2015, 2017, and 2018, respectively, with each one considered a box office success.

The kink community, however, was greatly displeased with the books and the subsequent movies for a variety of reasons but the most important one being that it depicted an unhealthy relationship with or without kink involved. In fact, despite the influx of newbies in sync with the various releases, those who profess to love any of the books or movies are often met with a sad shaking of the head and sometimes even presented with a discussion about how this franchise is a hindrance to the community.

The biggest issue that folks seem to have is that Mr. Grey (remember that from before?) is a stalker, obsessive, controlling, and quick to fly off the handle – all things repeatedly mentioned throughout the series and illustrated in the films. None of these traits are ones that anyone would want in a partner much less a dominant. Secondary issues with the overall story include there actually having very little kink and mostly sex with a controlling man, along with other things like Christian Grey is supposed to be an all-powerful business mogul who can negotiate or get whatever he wants yet he cannot get Anastasia to actually sign the contract throughout the entire first book, and his flip-flopping on things like saying he won't do anything with/to her until she signs yet he has sex with her without her signing anything.

The books and movies have been shredded in a slew of articles and reviews that you can look for online to give you far more detailed descriptions of the various issues with the writing, the production, the relationships, and the D/s dynamics. Suffice it to say, these books/movies are generally not well received by the community and should not be your expectation for what the lifestyle or a D/s dynamic is about in any way.

Real How-To Books

If you are going to spend your time reading it might as well be informative and written by people who actually know the lifestyle. If you start looking into "how to" kink books you'll start to see a few names over and over. Some of those folks include Jay Wiseman, Lee Harrington, Patrick Califia, Midori, Jack Rinella, and Dr. Gloria Brame. While I can't possibly name and go into all the books available by these authors and the countless others who have produced amazing works, I wanted to list a few that are good ones to start with for beginners. I've had the pleasure of meeting with Lee Harrington during one of his speaking engagements and a private meeting with him shortly after to help me learn more about being transgender and found his soft and comforting presence a big help to me in my personal journey as a trans person. I've also had the pleasure of getting to know Gloria Brame who is always engaging and continues to provide not just the kink community but society as a whole with many valuable resources as an esteemed sex therapist.

Joshua Tenpenny

- *Real Service*

Jack Rinella

- *Becoming a Slave: The Theory & Practice of Voluntary Servitude*
- *Complete Slave*
- *Partners in Power: Living in Kinky Relationships*

Robert J. Rubel

- *Protocols: A Variety of Views (Power Exchange Books Resource Series)*

Patrick Califia (Listed on the book as Pat Califia and sometimes listed as Patrick Califia-Rice)

- *Sensuous Magic: A Guide for Adventurous Lovers*

Lee Harrington

- *Playing Well with Others: Your Field Guide to Discovering, Exploring, and Navigating the Kink, Leather and BDSM Communities*
- *Sacred Kink*
- *Rope, Bondage, and Power – Power Exchange Books*

John Warren

- *The Loving Dominant*
- *Safe, Sane, Consensual and Fun*

Jay Wiseman

- *SM 101: A Realistic Introduction*

Philip Miller and Molly Devon

- *Screw the Roses, Send Me the Thorns: The Romance and Sexual Sorcery of Sadomasochism*

Dr. Gloria Brame

- *Different Loving: A Complete Exploration of the World of Sexual Dominance and Submission*

- *Different Loving Too: Real People, Real Lives, Real BDSM*

- *Come Hither: A Commonsense Guide to Kinky Sex*

Fiction

There are few books that depict BDSM in either a realistic or, at the very least, non-sleazy way. There are, however, a couple that I wanted to include.

Dr. Gloria Brame released her first fiction book *Champions of Pleasure* at the end of 2018. Brame brings her extensive experience with BDSM, sex, sexuality, and the insights into people through her various years being a board-certified sexologist to make the characters and situations come alive. One of the rare things this book does that so many others seem to fail at is to include a wide range of sexualities rather than the all-too-typical heterosexual couplings.

Additionally, I wanted to take a moment to include Jacqueline Carey's *Kushiel Legacy* series, most especially the Phedre Trilogy (the first three books). These books take place in a fantasy-esque version of our world and could be best described as being around the 12th century if we were to put a time period on it, although it's not a typical period piece. Nor is it a typical fantasy genre piece either but it does have that aura and there are some fantasy-realm elements. The language used throughout the books is awe-inspiring and for anyone who loves language and words, they will get immense pleasure from this series.

The reason I mention this series in a book regarding D/s and kink is that the lead character is, essentially, the perfect masochist and engaging in paid sessions for kink and sex is nothing out of the ordinary. Other than it not using kink as a lame excuse for a hot sex scene or as a cover for just being abusive it shows that sex and BDSM are not things of which to be ashamed. Further, these elements do not take over the entire plot but are rather beautiful accents to a well-woven story involving intricate relationships, court intrigue, murderous plots, and adventures all while learning about oneself.

Reality

Reality is very different from fiction whether you read it in a book or watch it in a movie or TV show. In this lifestyle, there needs to be an understanding and acceptance that no one is perfect, and both the submissive and dominant are bound to make mistakes. It can be a lot of work, as well, and not just physical work like doing chores but mental and emotional work as you both strive towards an exciting dynamic that continues to grow as you both learn and explore. There are going to be days when one or both of you just don't "feel like it" so you need to consider that ahead of time and have some options on how that will be handled specifically between you both. There are going to be days when it's just madness rushing around to do errands, deal with work, pay the bills, and all either of you wants to do is plop into bed and call it a day. There are going to be times when doing chores just sucks. Overall these things can be addressed and worked through with relative ease if you have good open communication habits and plan for them ahead of time.

There are ways to work your dynamic into nearly all aspects of your day whether you're together or apart and there are ways to make things fun and exciting. Being submissive to someone doesn't mean it has to be sad or feel bad because the entire point is to feel good and get the satisfaction (in whatever form) that you want from the experience. It can be fun and challenging, it can make you grow as a person, and it can be hot and thrilling. It can be whatever you both want it to be, but just go into things with a realization that it's not what Hollywood wants you to think.

SECTION TWO:
ONLINE COMMUNITY

The Internet is a great and powerful asset
as well as a short-cut to all things great and small.
It's a source of anonymity and a way to explore a vast
community without ever leaving the comfort of your own home.

Chapter 9

Protect Yourself

First and foremost – you are responsible for yourself and the actions you do or do not take. It doesn't matter that you're online and it's all seemingly anonymous. Yes, we're going to touch on a topic that seems to have fallen out of favor in our society and that is <u>personal responsibility</u>.

It is, without a doubt, a terrible thing to fall prey to scam artists as mentioned in a previous chapter, but they only succeed if you let them. One must be vigilant and maintain a certain level of common sense when engaged in **any** activity on the Internet, but most especially when we're talking about money and private information. It is your own personal duty to protect yourself. This isn't a victim-shaming scenario by any stretch of the imagination but rather it is a wake-up call that many online scams can be avoided with a little due diligence and – my favorite thing – common sense.

Nor is this intended to negate that, in fact, bad things do happen to the best of people regardless of what precautions are taken. Some scam artists have been at this a very long time and have learned the art of manipulation. While luckily a good number of scammers don't seem to be overly savvy, on occasion there's a true grifter in the mix. It still falls to you to be alert though, because (in most cases) there will be no one else there to protect you and tell you that the person you're speaking to is a scam artist or otherwise of ill repute.

Along these lines, however, are times when you may get a heads-up or words of caution and those should be given serious consideration. Sometimes a scam artist has made their way through enough people that the word spreads. Some people will put the username in their profile as a way to help warn others, some will make posts in messages boards, other times it may simply be word of mouth. If someone you're friends with online happens to see you're chatting with someone who has a bad or questionable reputation they may message you. Sometimes you will hear some scuttlebutt about someone to be leery of in person at events. Do take some of this with a grain of salt especially if it's an issue between them and only one other person. Use caution, but also consider that the gossip is just that, gossip, and likely being spread only to harm that person in a malicious way. However, if you hear some concerns or warnings raised about someone from a few different places it is, once again, best to avoid the potential situation entirely and focus your search efforts elsewhere.

To help you protect yourself, I want to focus primarily on online protection here as I will discuss some safety measures you can take once you go offline in another section.

Do Not Release Your Address: This should go without saying but, unfortunately, must be said because it's something that still happens. First and foremost, never put your specific location in your profile (yes, people actually do that). Do not exchange this information with someone after only a few chats online. In fact, you would be best advised to not even disclose it upon first meeting. If your chats go poorly or the first meeting is a bust, you don't want someone who could possibly be disgruntled to know where you live. Moreover, you don't want to give out your information and find out that the Domme's profile is fake. The person now has your name, can deduce your date of birth in most cases, and now has your address. Just don't do it. Save it for after you have a few meetings under your belt.

Be Aware: By honing your observational skills and trusting your gut you can navigate away from most of the scam artists. In fact, with enough practice, you can avoid them completely just by picking up on cues in their profile. Additionally, fine-tuning your observational skills on how people behave online and in real life can help you become a better submissive to your dominant as you are able to key-in to their needs and body language.

Trust Your Gut: As I said previously, your gut is incredibly important. Truly, if your other senses are overruling your desires and telling you that this seems far too good to be true then, in most cases, your intuition is right. While there's always that diamond in the rough or the real deal to be found, more often than not those warning bells are going off for a reason.

Who Can Access Your Information: Depending on what site or social networking forum you're using, there are often privacy settings to configure on who can and cannot access certain levels of information. While not all sites provide a wide selection of options, most will allow you to privatize your images. So as not to come off as someone unwilling to post a personal photograph or that all your pictures were scored from the Internet, you may want to consider a brief profile disclaimer like: "I have personal pictures set to friends only. I'd be happy to accept a friend request after we've chatted a bit." That means not posting any pictures that could be identifiable such as with your face or tattoos but that doesn't mean there should be no pictures – consider ones with your face cropped out or of your back.

Be aware that some sites may be indexed by search engines. There's at least one BDSM-related site that gives you the option to opt out of being searchable on popular search engines. Most dating websites, in general, do not allow their pages to be indexed in this manner but it is something to be aware of as a possibility because some do exist. If you're unsure about indexing feel free to contact the technical support team for whatever website you use.

Check the website to see if you can Right-click and/or Save Image As on pictures in people's profiles. Some will restrict this ability to help limit potential issues but there are always ways around those limits. While it's easy enough to do on a computer it's now extra-easy to bypass these limitation features on cell phones as it just takes a click of a button to make a screen cap. When posting pictures or personal details, even with privacy limitations, be aware that a screen cap is incredibly easy to do so only allow people you've developed a connection with access to these more identifiable pieces of your life.

Inviting Them to Non-Kink Social Networking Sites: Inviting new lifestyle acquaintances to view your family-friendly social networking pages can lead to problems. In some instances, pictures or comments have been posted that were inappropriate or unwanted on vanilla pages and have caused unnecessary stress, uncomfortable explanations, and struggles to get the images or comments removed. Sometimes it's not even done maliciously but rather what one person considers "no big deal" could be devastating to someone else if people in their vanilla life saw it.

The entire purpose of a kink social networking site is to avoid these types of exposures to the vanillas in our lives, so it's best to keep your other pages out of the equation until you're seriously involved with someone – in person in real life. As a small precaution, you can set up a secondary account on the vanilla pages that are dedicated only to your kink friends and activities. While it may be a little bit of a hassle juggling two Twitter or Instagram accounts, it's far less hassle than dealing with the issues if something risqué does get posted.

Hidden Information Made Public: There is a surprising amount of information that's embedded in nearly everything we do and a lot of it can make us traceable. While you don't have to be paranoid and never go online again, most people encountered online do not know about or have the know-how to access such information. It is important, however, to at least be aware of it yourself so you can take some steps to protect yourself.

One example is Geo-caching. This is a "tag" that's embedded into images taken by a cellphone and most cameras today. Due to the stalking and tracking risks that have developed, almost all devices now come with the option to turn the feature off but, in most cases, it is set "on" by default when you first get your device. While this feature is useful to photographers and photojournalists who want to mark the date, time, and location of the images they take, this is a key method of predators to locate you without you even realizing it. It's also a way to track your habits by seeing how often a particular location appears in the embedded information inside your pictures. This is a feature you will want to explore for your individual phone and possibly disconnect. In most instances when you upload images to a site, especially dating/kink-based, that information is not transferred and cannot be accessed by people who see the image on the website. It can still be made available on certain sites and social media platforms, however, so it's usually better to turn the feature off.

Check-in features on Facebook and other apps can be fun for some users. Most people don't actually care where you are and why you're there so this is actually more of an annoying thing people use for no purpose. Still, sites that do use it are often set to a public setting so anyone can see that you've checked in there. Even if your personal setting restricts that to be viewable only to friends the location you checked-in at may still have that showing up as public on their personal pages. While dating/kink sites do not typically have this feature on their own sites it's something to be aware of when you do it on your vanilla pages because that can be seen by other prying eyes who may want to find you off the dating/kink sites.

Friends/Circles: Friend requests are a special area for diligence. While it's nice to have a lot of friends on any social media forum including dating/kink sites and there's a sense of feeling popular, remember this can also work against you. Having an excessive number of "friends" can lead people viewing your profile to think that you're just a "collector" with little interest in anything more than increasing your numbers. On the other hand, too few could also indicate a socialization problem. Pick and choose your friends wisely. Once someone is a friend, they often have the ability to access your privatized details and if this is not really someone you trust with that information you need to keep them off your friend/circle list.

Who Can Access You: There is a relatively common practice that dominants will want the password to your various online accounts. This has proven to be an issue for new and seasoned players alike. This is something that should only be given out to someone with whom you have a clearly established, real-life relationship with and even then you may want to restrict that to only certain websites. That is, giving them your kink site password might be something you're comfortable with but not the login for your online banking pages. If you don't have a long established communication history **and** have met the person in real life a few times then do not give out your password. It's a hassle on many levels including getting technical support involved. Absolutely do not release passwords to vanilla accounts as the person can easily cause immeasurable damage before you can stop them. Plus, you need to consider that the moment they have your password they can change it to something else and never let you know what it is so getting in touch with technical support to stop them from ruining your life could become incredibly difficult.

Avoid the issue entirely and just do not give out your account information. Not every dominant wants this information but if you come across someone who wants it after only a few emails back and forth then that's a red flag. If you tell them that you won't give them the passwords and they get nasty, abusive, or manipulative about it that's all you need to know that this person is probably up to no good and your best course of action is to just move on to someone else.

Additionally, don't be fooled into using tracking software and apps. The software can be hidden in file attachments and are usually known as keyloggers so be wary when downloading files from people you're only just starting contact with and use caution when allowing them access to GPS tracking apps through your online accounts and phone apps. While you can usually deny access or remove the app you may forget they even have access to it. This also includes online calendars and online server accesses (such as the cloud where someone can access your email, calendars, and contacts).

What NOT to Include: I have come across profiles in a geographical search (such as for my nearby area) that have included full names. On most sites, there is an automatic birth date or age that will display. With a quick online search based on your full name, age, and general location odds are pretty good that someone can find the real you. Furthermore, never put your phone number in your profile. While cell phones are a little harder to pinpoint using reverse number searches it's absolutely possible to do. Make an email address without your real name used in the sign-up process or anywhere in the email address itself. Also, do not use birthdate related numbers in your email address or any of your usernames.

Get A Scene Name: Pick a name that is easy for people to shorten and use aloud without revealing or using your real name. Footboy1234 doesn't allow for many other options than someone shouting, "Hey footboy!" from across a room. While most lifestylers will be talking to you in email or at lifestyle-type events, you could be meeting at a restaurant or other public place so give careful consideration as to what you want to be called. Some people feel comfortable enough with using their first name when meeting people as it is still difficult to track someone with only a first name, while others do not want anyone knowing anything private about them. This will be a personal judgment call you will have to make.

Do Not Release Financial Details: Finances are a very touchy and personal subject. For those seeking a real-life relationship, this topic will inevitably come up but shouldn't come into play until much further down the road after many personal engagements. It is best to speak in broad terms such as, "I'm employed, I manage my bills, I won't be a financial burden," or similar statements. This is, actually, something a real-life dominant will want and need to know if they're going to consider you for a live-in or serious real-life situation. If someone is employed or not, for example, is important for both sides to know as that can be a deciding factor if things make it to a real-life/long-term status.

Most dominants do not want to be the sole financial provider and many are happy with splitting expenses, but they want to know that this is something you're actually capable of doing before investing a lot of time and energy into a potential relationship. Disclosing your annual salary (or range) is a question found on many public surveys or applications so it is really a matter of personal comfort as to whether or not you disclose that information. What you may want to do, especially in the beginning, is maintain the use of broad terms saying things like, "I receive retirement benefits," or "I only work part-time because I'm in school full-time." These statements don't give too much away while indicating that you have your own income source and aren't looking to freeload.

**Remember, information put on the Internet
is permanent, even if you think you deleted it.**

Tattoos/Scars: Ink is very sexy! Many take significant pride in the work they've had done and love to show it off. Remember, however, that your tattoos are identifiable characteristics. For a fairly public profile, you may want to blur out some of the work, especially if it's a unique piece. Scars can be a mixed bag as they can be both identifiable and yet fairly generic. Many scars look alike, seeing a scar will not necessarily immediately out you, but if there's just enough information about you plus an identifiable scar it could be enough for someone to figure out who you are in real life.

Your History Can Be Tracked: This can work in your favor in two ways. On most sites, when a person checks out your profile they can see if you're a member of any discussion groups or what your previous posting history has been. Benefit number one is that this can provide a potential dominant a great deal of insight into who you are, how you can handle a discussion, and how easily you get riled up. This can also work against you. If your posts tend to fly off the handle, be poorly written, off-topic, or generally juvenile this will reflect poorly on you. The second benefit is the feature works both ways. You can follow what the dominant has been posting just as easily in order to learn about their interests and see how they behave online to get a better feel for how they interact with people. Do they get uppity at the drop of a hat? Do they demand absolute submission from everyone without cause? Do they integrate well with the conversation and provide good and sound insights? Use forums and discussion boards to sell yourself by simply being you. Be careful in your posts, use manners, and lay a trail that you are proud to have seen and not something you'll want to hide from or have to defend later.

Also, be aware that some websites have features where just clicking on the person's profile will show them that you visited. In most cases being a visitor to someone's profile is no big deal – that's how we determine if it's worth messaging someone or not. However, if you message someone and then visit their profile every single day while you await a response it could be pretty creepy. Visiting someone's profile repeatedly, especially in a short timespan without messaging them at all could be equally creepy. Some sites, however, allow "premium" members to view profiles in stealth mode so just because you haven't seen them appear in your visitor log doesn't mean they haven't actually seen your profile.

Reverse Image Search: This is another double-edged sword and I've already discussed how it can be used to find fake profiles but this is how it can also be used against you. Remember, just as you can search, you can be searched. If you're using any images on both your vanilla pages (like social media accounts) as you use on your kinky profile, then someone may be able to reverse image search your picture and find the real you or, at least, find your other online accounts and try to reach out to you there or try to keep digging to find you in person. It's recommended that you perform these searches on your own images periodically to see where your pictures may have been posted without your knowledge. First, it will help you determine if you can be easily located, and second, it can help you discover if someone has stolen your image.

Unfortunately, there is no magic formula to identify people who are up to no good, whether to bilk you out of your money, blackmail you or randomly disrupt your life. Minor incidents could be considered a life lesson as you become more adept at spotting these unsavory people by actually encountering them. Hopefully you will avoid any major issues, and the best way to do that is to be aware of what's possible and some ways to protect yourself.

Remember that there are tools and resources available by typing in a few simple keywords. Don't shun this often untapped source of information... the Internet. Many use it blindly to make the connections they want but never harness the power of the Web to learn about vitally important issues such as Internet Safety, current scams, or verifying profile pictures. Use the full scope of the tools available and quickly learn to navigate through and around those with ill-intent.

Chapter 10

Profile Pictures – Classy or Just Gross?

This is actually something that occurs with surprising regularity and thus warrants a chapter all on its own. First and foremost, anyone who creates a profile on a BDSM social networking/dating site needs to be aware that their main profile picture (or avatar) will be *the* first thing a dominant will see. Whether you're emailing a dominant for the first time, they see posts you're making in forums, or they're scrolling through profiles at random, most sites are designed to show your avatar right next to your name. This is your first impression regardless of how it is found, so make it the best impression possible.

Remember, a picture speaks a thousand words.

First, take a moment to explore the site you're on and get a feel for the general theme. If you're on a site that caters primarily to sexual hookups with little interest in establishing significant relationships then go buck-wild with naked and sexually suggestive/explicit pictures. However, if you're on a site that caters more toward making personal connections with people (which is what this book focuses on accomplishing), a closeup picture of your genitals shouldn't necessarily be the first impression you're making.

Remember, many sites are designed so that every single post you make, whether it's in a forum, chat, or status update, your avatar is stamped right there next to it. Many dominants (even if they're big fans of sexy pictures) don't want their walls or feeds inundated with boobs, cocks, asses and such, especially if they're in a lengthy email or chat sessions with you. Over and over again I see responses from dominants, particularly women, stating emphatically that seeing a person with any genitals as their avatar is more of a turn-off than a turn-on. They also often see it as saying, "this is all I have to offer you," or "this is the most important part of me," and that's the last thing most dominants are looking for, especially if they're seeking a long-term connection. They want to see that you care about something other than your body or just getting yourself off.

Having no avatar at all is equally troubling. While almost anyone on a BDSM-related site will understand that many need privacy or absolute discretion, there's really little need to be completely without an image of some kind. A shot that shows you, but with your face blurred, or even cropped out entirely, can still be helpful. It gives someone an immediate idea as to your general physique, how you present yourself, and even your style.

Are you a…

- Punk rocker?

- Business person?

- Laid back average Joe?

- A complete slob?

The complete absence of a picture could be a red flag as it says many different things about you. It could be that you're uncomfortable or unhappy with your own physical appearance, you feel that your necessary level of discretion requires absolute anonymity, or you're just simply too lazy to be bothered. Many dominants will assume one or all of those things are true and most simply will not initiate or respond to any messages from no-picture profiles. In fact, many sites give the option that those without an image be excluded from search results so you, right off the bat, are out of the running entirely. Laziness is the opposite attitude you want to project as a potential submissive, and deceit is not the proper approach to take in meeting a dominant.

As much as you want to display only your most awesome qualities and then eventually easing into any less favorable attributes, you need to actually balance this approach. If a dominant isn't looking for or interested in you – the good, bad, and ugly – then they aren't someone you need to be wasting your time trying to pursue. As the saying goes: "There are plenty of other fish in the sea." Remember, the entire point of your search isn't just to hook up with a dominant, but to specifically find a dominant with whom you're *compatible* so that you can work toward a long-term dynamic.

Assuming now that you have an acceptable avatar and a dominant wants to investigate further, it doesn't mean you can move all your genital shots into the rest of your profile or album(s). Having one acceptable photo as an avatar and the rest of your pictures showing your genitals is just as tasteless and once more screams that getting your sexual pleasure is all you think about. I cannot emphasize this enough or tell you how often this *exact* topic comes up in discussions between dominants of all genders and sexualities. This doesn't mean you can't have any sexual pictures in your profile. By all means, include a few, but do not let them be the only ones, your avatar, or otherwise overwhelm your profile.

Kinky Does Not Mean Tasteless

While this shouldn't need saying, unfortunately… it does. Stay away from anything that can look creepy. Holding a weapon of any kind, especially as a submissive, is extremely not recommended. If you thoroughly enjoy knife-play, get a friend who is willing to have at least an arm/hand in the shot use it in some *erotic* manner that could appeal to a dominant who enjoys knife-play as well. Try to include an image that has you at least basically well-groomed. Watch out for making creepy faces like snarls, and that could include grimaces of pain that just don't translate well in the picture. Also, watch out for making funny or silly faces as they, too, do not always translate well in pictures. If in doubt take it out – that is, if you have to consider if the picture seems creepy, the best option is to leave it out entirely. The point is to make your pictures reflect the real you, and not seem like mug shots.

It's surprising that the need to mention not making crazy faces, extremely wide and bulging eyes, snarling facial expressions, or anything else that could in some way be creepy or scary is necessary, but there are far too many profiles out there with those exact issues. This is especially concerning for male submissives seeking female dominants as the last thing a woman wants in their life is someone who looks psychotic. Having someone who looks psychotic in an ambiguous online album is not alluring, sexy, or erotic in any way and is **certainly** not someone a dominant (especially a female) would ever consider being alone with in their home, much less anywhere near their body, without an army of people between them.

Lastly, don't have an entire album dedicated to comics, drawings, or any other photographs that were clearly taken from the web and especially porn sites. And, under no circumstances, ever – and I mean never ever – should you post pictures of others. Nor should you ever claim to own images that are not yours and that includes by allusion or outright.

- It tells everyone you're dishonest. Since honesty and trustworthiness are imperative in this lifestyle, anyone who is dishonest over a simple thing like the copyright of an image means they can't be trusted with major things like playing safe.

- It shows that you're likely a player with no real intention (or imagination for that matter). Those who do this are typically more interested in scavenging the web for images they think are cool or turn them on and living the fantasy of it in their head rather than actually doing anything about it in real life.

- You will more than likely get caught and called out on it and could easily get into copyright infringement trouble. Yes, it is illegal to take someone else's hard work and claim it as your own. Even if the copyright owner doesn't take action against you many websites will not tolerate it and you could find your account/profile restricted, temporarily disabled, or permanently banned.

If there is a picture, comic, or image you find that really calls to your passion, by all means, use it. A couple of these are fine, especially if you haven't gained the real-life experience to have your photo taken in a similar scenario but really want to express your interest in the topic. However, state clearly where you got it, who owns the copyright, and that it's not you in the photo but that you find the subject matter thrilling or intriguing. It's not always easy to find who owns the copyright (even if you use Reverse Image Search) so simply putting a statement like: "Not sure whose picture this is but I really liked it because…" and even adding, "If you know who owns the picture please let me know so I can add the citation," would actually go a long way in your favor. It shows you're honest, you care about the work others do, you are respectful, and you are willing to correct something if necessary.

There is a current trend to inundate profiles (those with unlimited album space) with memes (pronunciation: sounds like creams – not me-me). In fact, many will display these as their public images. While this, in itself, is fine, it is vital to have personal images that, once you've become friends, the dominants can see. It's helpful to still have at least one 'public' image of yourself visible even if it's cropped or blurred. Just as you shouldn't have genital pictures be the bulk of your content, memes shouldn't be either.

I do want to include a cautionary word about memes. Remember that they, too, will provide insight as to the type of person you are. If they are all snarky, snide, obnoxious, or 'in your face,' this could tell a prospective dominant that you're confrontational and that you're not looking for a power exchange, but rather a power struggle. Most of us can appreciate a good dose of sarcasm, so don't be afraid to use humor, but if vicious sarcasm is the recurring theme, most dominants will pass.

Further, political or religious memes can be a sticky situation. It can work either for you or against you. Politics and religion are amongst the most delicate of subjects and opposing sides will often be very adamant in their views. Making your political and religious opinions known in writings on your profile or with the use of memes can help weed out dominants who feel they cannot be with someone with your particular viewpoint, and it may also lure in ones who share your opinions giving you some common ground with which to start. Just be aware, however, that it could also make you susceptible to "attacks" from those of oppositional standpoints. You do not have to engage with them, especially if it's in message boards or other more public areas. Engaging in a battle like this where potential dominants could see your posts at any time (as we already covered) could work against you, not to mention that these battles almost never end with anyone changing their minds on the subject. Just report the harassment to the moderator or the site owner and go on about your day.

Stay away from hate-memes as many sites will not allow any form of hate speech. This is a topic that has gained a lot of attention in recent years and continues to be considered a security issue. Many sites will remove the image(s) without warning, may inform you that the image(s) were deleted, or may even suspend or terminate your account. Hate speech in some countries is illegal, and many websites' Terms of Service (TOS)/Terms of Use (TOU) will expressly forbid images or wording that could be construed as inciting hate. While you have the right to freedom of expression about almost anything you want, other users have the right to use the site without worrying about hate speech.

While there are bigots in all aspects of our world (including the lifestyle), the kink community is one of the most open-minded, tolerant and inclusive communities you will find. If your kink includes things like Race/Nazi-play or if you like to be spoken to in a degrading way, having your race, religion, gender, or sexuality used against you, then it's best to explain that in writing inside your profile and not through the use of memes. Explaining in your profile that you're interested in any of these things being a part of your dynamic (or sessions) is fine, as long as it is not worded in such a way that it comes off more like hate speech than explaining your kink.

Chapter 11

The Art of Profile Writing

*S*ince the intent of this book is to help you find a dominant that you want to serve, I'm going to ignore the sites/apps out there designed for cybering, sex hook-ups, and other non-relationship purposes.

Whether a dominant happens to scroll through profiles (yes, it does happen), whether you caught their attention through posting in forums, or you initiated contact through email and they want to check your profile before responding – it doesn't matter how they come to be at your profile, they are there. What is important now is what your profile says, how it 'sounds' or comes across, and the 'image' you're projecting. You need to have a nice balance of information, without confessing everything. It has to be understandable and concise without ranting or rambling. It needs to explain who you are a bit as a person and as a submissive (especially explaining if you're experienced or new), what you're looking for, and even what you're not looking for. There needs to be *something* of worth there.

It's possible you sent a fantastic email that made the dominant want to respond, but when they visit your profile, and you can pretty much guarantee that they will, if it's blank, sparse, poorly written, or screams "obnoxious," chances are great that your email will be deleted with all the rest, no matter how wonderful and unique it was.

One major thing **NOT** to do is leave your profile blank or write something like, "I just signed up/don't know what to write and will get to this part later." If you are finding the time to peruse dominant profiles and send out emails, you should have used that time for a better purpose such as developing your profile. This is absolutely putting the cart before the horse and it's a major thing to avoid. It will almost always guarantee your email is deleted without response. Also, some sites allow users to see when you joined (or how many days you've been a member), so if your profile still says that you will get to your profile-writing a month later, you look full-of-it or just plain lazy and we already covered the issue with being perceived as lazy.

We all understand that creating a profile can be daunting as it requires time and some considerable thought about one's self. However, it's also one of the first impressions you're going to make regardless of the fabulousness of your emails. Being able to look into yourself will be an ongoing thing you experience as a submissive and to be embraced. It doesn't have to take you hours to write, it doesn't have to be several pages in length. It does, however, have to contain something and should include some of the basics mentioned above.

Using some humor and witticism in your writing is encouraged, but it should be used sparingly. Remember that those reading your profile cannot see your facial expressions or "hear" the tone of your voice, so some of your charms may be lost or even come across as sarcastic or generally obnoxious. Since the person reading your profile doesn't know anything about you, they don't yet understand your particular brand of humor and may misread your comedic approach as offensive. Don't be afraid to use some levity, the lifestyle is not all about being stoic and serious, but just use some caution in how you use it. Balance out the sense of humor with genuine content because this is your profile, not your cheat-sheet for a stand-up act. Also, even if you think it's funny, do not joke about serious matters or current hot topics or general touchy subjects like politics and religion.

Make sure it's readable. That means making sure your spelling, grammar, and sentence structure are clear and correct. If English is not your native language or you have a disability that makes writing difficult, then make sure you put that in at the top of your profile. Making sure it's right up front allows someone reading your profile the option to give you leeway on any mistakes because of these issues rather than assuming other more negative-type things. You can write your profile in a document, such as MS Office or OpenOffice, where you have the option to see any spelling mistakes. Using most browsers today also gives you the option to have a little red line show up under a word that's misspelled. Something like Grammarly can be used for free and has the option to be downloaded to Windows computers, installed on to browsers, or installed for use with Word. It provides you with a much more comprehensive spellcheck and sentence structure tools and is completely free to use as much as you want. While you don't have to write like a doctoral candidate, it is important that you still express yourself clearly.

Regardless of what option you take, be sure to re-read your profile. In fact, read it out loud or use a reader program to have it read to you (including some cell phone features that will read content on the screen). If you stumble over it then surely someone else will. Additionally, you may have spelled a word correctly but it may be the wrong word. While programs like Grammarly will often detect this as being a mistake, nothing is foolproof and it's something that can easily be missed if you don't use such a program.

FOR EXAMPLE:

"My goat is to serve a dominant long-term." Goat is a word that is spelled correctly but is definitely not the word you intended. MS Office and Grammarly will both pick up this error although Office doesn't always catch these mistakes.

Do note, however, that certain words we use in the lifestyle are "errors" in most programs. FemDom, submissives, slashy-speak or lower case on submissive-based words and upper on dominant-based words throughout a sentence will show as needing correction.

Use a period, question mark, and exclamation point to end a sentence and not a comma. Furthermore, use only one form of punctuation unless you are purposefully using an ellipse (…) the occasional - ?!? - for emphasizing alarm and/or confusion. For no other reason should you use multiple periods, commas, or question marks in a row.

FOR EXAMPLE:

Dear Mistress,,, i found your profile interesting., would you be interested in talking,,, i'd love to hear back from you,,,

I received emails and passed countless profiles written exactly in that way. While the overall content is a close replication of the inane emails many of us receive, it's worsened by the atrocious punctuation. As you can see, the quality (or rather the lack thereof) of emails we get can very well make us jaded, and this is just one reason why it's so difficult to find a match. The moment we see a message in a format like this, we hit the delete button. However, there are some dominants – especially if you caught them on a bad day – who will be more than happy to send you a response that is harsh ridicule of a message such as this. The moment we come upon a profile written in this manner, we're gone. We're off that profile just as fast as we clicked on it and on to reading someone else's who has some basic understanding of writing.

A good way to think of your profile, especially when making sure it contains proper spelling and grammar, is that it is like a first date. You wouldn't show up for a date (with anyone, not just with a dominant) unwashed, in dirty jeans, rumpled shirt or skirt/dress, and sloppy hair. Your profile is your first introduction, so think of it as your first date and make sure it's nice and neat.

Conversely, you don't want to sound like you're writing a resume or that you're the best thing since sliced bread. We can all be good at things but if your profile comes off as overly-pompous, we're just going to opt out. By all means, write intelligently and tell us how much you love the Opera or that you have tons of degrees or certifications. We love educated people. We just don't like it when people act entitled. Do you have a Master's degree in Physics? That's awesome. The dominant you're emailing, or wanting to speak with, could have a Ph.D. in Quantum Physics – but if you come across sounding like a snob or, better yet, that you know more than they do, they will not tolerate it. If you are a male speaking to a female, whatever you do, **do not** mansplain. As I've said, we enjoy intelligence, we even like some intellectual discourse or a fun debate, and we do – contrary to what porn would like you to think – like speaking to our submissives. But we're not going to speak to someone who is belittling or demeaning in the manner of their speech. Submissive doesn't mean dumb, but it does mean humble. Modesty, in general, is a pleasant character trait regardless of how you identify.

There are no rules (but there are some guides, such as this book) on how short or long a profile should be and it comes down to your best judgment. One thing you should stay away from is an extremely short profile, especially one that has virtually no information, quotes only, or is just a list of your kinks. Again, absolutely refrain from your entire profile consisting of statements like:

- My name says it all.

- I'm new so I'll get to this later.

- I never know to write in these things, I'm just looking for a dominant.

- New and looking to learn.

- Anything you want to know, just ask me.

- I am a total submissive and I want a dom.

These little "gems" have **_all_** been seen on profiles and not just one or two that pop up sporadically. These are *common* profile statements and often the only content in the entire profile field. Do not write a few lines and then five pages worth of quotes either. While the occasional quote can be inspiring and can provide some enlightenment to the reader as to the type of person you may be, inundating a profile with quotes is an utter waste of time. Several kink sites have a journal or blog option. Put your quotes there and save the profile field for – you guessed it – information about yourself.

Extra-long profiles should be done carefully. While they are not necessarily a bad thing, you should pay attention to what is being said. Are you just reiterating the same thing or are you genuinely sharing details? Are you complaining about all your bad experiences in the lifestyle or talking about yourself and your interests? While you shouldn't be writing a whole book about your life you do want to include key details, especially things that may be major turn-offs or deal breakers for you (or even things you like that may be an issue for someone else – like race-play as mentioned above) or include things about the type of person/relationship you are seeking. Besides, you don't want to put everything you can think of about you and your interests in kink and vanilla all in the profile or you won't have much to talk about during the emails.

Remember, however, that the more specific you make your search, the more difficult it becomes. If your profile is a virtual dissertation on what you must have and what you absolutely don't want, then you are potentially missing out on meeting someone who may not fit into that small little box you created but could wind up being the best person for you. While there's no need to compromise there should be a level of open-mindedness as well.

The point of the profile is to tell others about yourself - as a person - not to publish a shopping list of your kinks and what you expect the dominant who gets you to do for you. It shouldn't be demanding in tone, saying things like, "My Dominant should be this type of person," or "My ideal Dominant will do this and that." It's abrasive, off-putting, and obnoxious. It says you're a Do-Me type who really only wants to get what they want with little to no consideration for the other person. If your profile is like this, you may want to just stop seeking a partner and head over to the local professional dominant. The 'tone' is very important in a profile, which is why I previously mentioned using humor with caution. As important as the tone is, it is also very difficult to express when using just the written word. A good rule of thumb is to write when you're in a specific mood. If you're going for fun and upbeat, then write when you're in a great mood. If you're going for calm and controlled, do some yoga or meditation before writing. Alternatively, do not write your profile while you're upset about anything. The mindset you have while writing will often be conveyed subconsciously into the words you choose or the way you phrase your sentences.

While listing some kinks that you really desire in your profile is okay, it's important to not come across as demanding, topping from the bottom, or wheedling. In fact, kink listing is discussed in a separate chapter as it's a frequent issue handled differently by various sites.

If you are affiliated with any groups in your area, including munches, you should include a few of them in your profile. These should be active memberships you hold to real-life groups and events you attend, not just groups located in your area that you've never been to or went to once a long time ago. Also, if you happen to actually be a member of a lot of groups you don't have to list them all, just a couple is fine for people to get a basic idea. You can simply state the name of the group/munch with which you are affiliated but, if you want, some sites will allow you to include a link to the group/munch site (if there is one). This helps illustrate to someone that you are active in the community, exploring the lifestyle, and to a certain extent taking the lifestyle seriously. While affiliations are not required, and not being known in the community doesn't mean you don't take the lifestyle seriously, it does help paint a better picture to a dominant. Alternatively, such information on a dominant's profile will tell you about their level of engagement and interests as well.

As far as groups go, I am speaking specifically about gatherings that take place off the Internet and require you to actually go somewhere and interact with people in a real-world setting. Being a member of 75 discussion groups does not count. Almost anyone can join any discussion group or forum, it does not require actual interaction (i.e. you can be a lurker), and while it does give someone a sense of what your interests are, it does nothing to say that you're interested in real-world interaction.

What else should you include in your profile? Here are some things to consider:

- How about those long walks on the beach? Or, do you hate the sand? Are you afraid of the water? Do you hate long walks in general? If you love the beach – what do you like about it? How often do you get to go? Is it to the ocean, bay, lakes?

- Are you a professional of some kind? If so, can you mention anything about it, even in broad terms, that could be interesting without giving away too much personal information?

- Are you a student? If so, what are you studying? When do you expect to be done with school? Once you're done would you be able to relocate for the right situation?

- Do you travel a lot? If so, is it for work or pleasure? Any places you go to more than others?

- Are you an avid fan of something? Books? TV/movies? Cycling? Boxing? Knitting?

- Do you have a unique or helpful skill? Massage therapy? Computer skills? Handyman? Cooking/baking? Not just things that you like or think you could pull off – but things that you are actually skilled at doing.

- How can your knowledge, education, work, or skills be a benefit to a dominant?

- Is there something that you're terrified of? Not necessarily a hard limit, but something, in general, that is a major fear that a potential dominant should know about?

- Ask some friends how they would describe you and apply some of that information.

- Do you have a dream or aspiration – no matter how big or small, something very important to you and you'd like your dominant to allow or possibly even be involved in?

- You can go generic and list/talk about some "favorites" like your favorite book/author, movie, TV show, animal, color, etc.

- Do you have role models or personal heroes? Who are they and why?

Think of questions you'd want to ask someone else and then answer them for yourself as a way to help fill your profile and shed some light on the type of **person** (not just submissive) you are. You can even search for "good questions for a profile" or similar terms and use them as a good jumping off point.

Further, you should be honest about your level of experience. If you have multiple years just milling around in the lifestyle but haven't really done many scenes or served anyone, have served one or even multiple dominants, have just played casually, or you're just starting out – any of these things should be made clear in your profile. A lack of experience is not necessarily a bad thing as many dominants see it as an opportunity to school someone fresh without previous training getting in the way. However, some prefer a submissive with experience so they don't have to start from scratch and the submissive will have a better idea of what they're comfortable exploring.

The most important piece of advice here, beyond saying you really do need to fill it out, is to keep it honest and enlightening without being overwhelming. And, whatever you do, stay away from being creepy. Take your time, write it out in Word or a similar program, spellcheck it, and remember to be yourself. A good exercise is to read through several other profiles before you start yours so that you can get an idea of things to include and see examples of what not to do in your own profile.

Chapter 12

Fetish/Kink Lists

Accessing fetish checklists, researching some of the terms, or just seeing what's out there can help you learn more about what does and doesn't interest you. There are countless times I've looked up a fetish that I saw on someone's profile and found it was a hard limit or, alternatively, something I thought I'd actually enjoy. In fact, this is a great way to initiate a conversation, especially if you're genuinely looking to learn about the lifestyle. If you see someone has a particular fetish or set of kinks that you're unsure of, you can email them to ask about their experience. Researching the term online is advised before you do this so you can ask intelligent questions and not seem like you're trolling for something. Learning about the experiences of others may broaden your mind more than reading a bland description or definition. That is, don't email someone asking, "What is x, y, z," when it would take just a second to look it up yourself. Instead, ask something like: "I saw you're interested in x, y, z. I'm pretty new to the lifestyle and this sounds like something I may be interested in, could you share a little about your experience in it so I can learn a little more about it?"

Most sites will allow you to select, check mark, add, or even create all kinds of fetishes which can become a rather substantial list while other sites restrict this to just a handful of kinks that you can select options for such as if you've done it, not done it, or if it's a limit. In either case, you may even come across some you have to look up as they may use the more technical term such as **dacryphilia** – an interest or arousal from being made to cry/making someone cry. Other terms could be those used often enough in the lifestyle but you may not know the term if you're new or just don't have an interest in those areas. A good example of this would be **bastinado** which is punishment or torture to the soles of someone's feet. It's just as easily referred to as <u>**foot whipping**</u> but will more often be called bastinado.

Some sites give you the opportunity to explore endless fetish lists which could include ones that are pretty much the same thing but just have a small word or spelling variation. Since some sites will allow you to create your own fetish, some listings could seem completely random or rare or some that are even whimsical and have absolutely nothing to do with kink or those that are focused on a specific person or event. There may be an option to declare from what perspective you enjoy the kink (i.e. dominant/submissive), if you're into or just curious about it, like to watch others do/wear it or like to do/be watched.

Unfortunately, there is no one site known at this time that includes the ability to clarify the extent, level, or experience in all of these ways but typically the sites do provide enough options to give you a good chance to express your interests. On my website (my contact information is at the end of this book), there is a comprehensive checklist of kinks that continues to be a work in progress. If you really want to be gung-ho about your fetishes you are welcome to use the checklist as a guide.

Many dominants will peruse these lists to get a general idea of what you enjoy. If you have a substantial list (and it can easily become so) chances are the person checking your fetishes will just skim through them for a quick idea and will not read every single one. In fact, unless they're actively "perving your list" to increase their own list of fetishes, chances are extremely rare that anyone will actually read through each and everyone you have. Alternatively, it's a good idea to go through other profiles to see what people have listed that may sound interesting or something you want to look up to learn about in further detail.

When put on the spot with questions like: "So what do you like," it's really easy to suddenly draw a blank or to list just a couple of things that are the more common fetishes. Having lists like this can be a great help to both learn more about the lifestyle as you encounter things you've not heard of before and as a way of expressing yourself as you list things that you would like to experience within your dynamic. It is important, however, to be realistic and not put 'craves bullwhip' if you've never experienced a whipping. Certain things, like whippings, can be very intense and the real feelings they create can be not at all what your fantasy expected. If you've never experienced a whip of any kind but the idea thrills you then it's okay to put "curious about" or "would like to try" next to the fetish.

It's very easy to get lost down the rabbit hole when it comes to fetish lists, especially on certain websites that allow you a virtually inexhaustible list. When you're first getting established, however, it's best to avoid duplications. You do not need to include eight different variations of biting as it becomes redundant and will often result in someone moving on without noticing your other interests. It's okay to add a few similar ones with the intention of trimming them shortly thereafter because it is easier to add and delete than go hunting through the masses again for that specific one that tickled your fancy. It's even okay to leave a few similar ones in your lists if it's really something you're passionate about and there's enough variation in each listing. While it's also okay to leave a million duplicated fetishes, it's typically not advised since, as I mentioned, it will bore someone quickly and they will leave your profile and likely miss seeing something that would have been a great fetish to connect you together. Let your list grow organically as you establish your reputation rather than inundate it right from the start.

This is your moment to indulge in your fetishes and get the word out there. This is where you can/want to list everything your heart desires (check the site's TOU for their policy on listing things they consider taboos including things like race play). Since some sites have designated areas specifically for fetish listings anyone who enters/scrolls to that area knows, without a doubt, they are going to see nothing but kinks and that's the express purpose of going there.

Other sites that have limited options for adding fetishes may mean you have to put them inside the profile content area. Only put fetishes in the profile area if there are no other options or the options available are very limited. If you have to put it in the profile content area then put it after the main portion of your profile, toward the bottom. It wouldn't be a bad thing if you were to add a little disclaimer that you're adding these fetishes here because the site is too limited. Do not, however, have the fetishes be the only thing in your profile content area. Furthermore, do not list every fetish you can think of in this area. Since it's in the main profile area try to narrow it down to just the ones that mean the most to you, avoid duplicates or slight variations of the same fetish, and keep it in one area, not spread throughout the whole profile. Whenever possible, if the site offers a journal/blog type of feature, it's recommended that you put fetish lists in those areas and make a brief mention in your profile along the lines of: "To see the different kinds of fetishes I really enjoy please check out my journal," and some sites will even allow you to link directly to that specific entry.

In many cases, you can save the list (such as the one on my website - my contact information is at the end of this book) or bookmark/favorite the page or profile that has fetishes you really enjoy so you can go back to them whenever you want, as often as you want. This is especially a good idea as certain sites will show up in your friends' wall feed each and every time you do anything, including every fetish added, and this could easily get you unfriended, unfollowed, or just generally be annoying to your friends. If you want to add tons of fetishes on sites that operate this way then do it in bursts of 10-15 fetishes a day and maybe not do it every single day. However, if you're new and don't have any friends/followers now is the time to go all out and add everything you want since you won't be infringing on anyone at this point. Also, saving and going back to the list periodically will help your sanity.

As I mentioned, it's easy to get lost in listing and learning about all kinds of fetishes but don't let it overwhelm you either. This part of your profile should be fun for you and others. Also, remember that your interests will change over time as you learn and grow within the lifestyle. In fact, it's a good idea to return to those links, profiles, or checklists periodically to see if something you were disinterested in before is now something you're curious about or if something you thought was a must-have fetish turned out to be not your thing. Just because it's there in a list or on your profile doesn't mean it's set in stone.

Before creating your own fetish or kink item (as some sites allow) you should be diligent in checking to see if something like that already exists. It's always better to opt into an existing fetish rather than make a duplicate. That means you may have to look for fetishes by their 'technical' term. As I mentioned earlier, having to look up a term isn't a bad thing and sometimes something that sounds scary or foreign may well be something you are interested in and just happens to be known by another name.

Do not have a decent list of fetishes in the fetish section and then just repeat them in the profile content area – whether you have a great profile or the fetishes are the only thing you post. Duplicating the fetishes in multiple areas can indicate that you're desperate to experience these fetishes and while that's important to you (and a major point to the lifestyle in general), it doesn't always give you the positive spin you think it might. While plastering your fetishes in every part of your profile that you can squeeze them into will definitely tell a dominant that you're very interested in a variety of things, it also says that experiencing your fetishes is the only thing you're interested in and not necessarily interested in being in a long-term D/s dynamic.

Remember, as I mentioned in the beginning, there are kinksters and fetishists and there's absolutely nothing wrong with being either of those. The only thing is that they are typically not looking to be in a D/s dynamic and specifically not one that will be long-term. Since the point of this book is to help you find the dominant who you want to serve in a D/s dynamic, you want to make sure you stay away from things like painting your profile to be that of someone interested in just fetish exploration rather than someone seeking to serve. Fetish exploration is a fun thing to do and it will often be done as you make your way through the local scene or with the dominant you are looking to serve.

In a D/s dynamic it's important that the submissive have their needs met just as much as the dominant has theirs satisfied, so finding a dominant into as many of the same fetishes you have is definitely an important thing. Having these lists, no matter how great or small, can be a big help in weeding out the dominants who don't enjoy them so you can narrow your searches to those who would be most compatible. It's just as important to also understand that the 'tone' of a profile at first glance is perhaps the most important step as it will often be the thing that will determine if a dominant emails/responds to you.

Chapter 13

Tech It Out

There are plenty of sites and apps available to use to help in your search whether it's for writing a better profile, kink-dedicated sites, or apps to help you chat and stay in touch. As with anything these days, there are some that remain through the years, some that are slowly losing ground, and some that blaze on to the scene only to fizzle out soon after. Here we will cover a little of everything but realize that while I try to keep the book current there are bound to be resources that have been phased out or have lessened in popularity.

Vanilla

There is a multitude of vanilla-based dating sites and apps and some have even gained such immense popularity that they've become part of our pop culture and lexicon. However, while they are primarily intended for and targeted to vanilla dating, there are still a variety of profiles out there for kinky people. The typical dynamic in these instances is either to be a more vanilla type of relationship with some kink in the bedroom or maintaining a traditional-seeming relationship with kink being a primary foundation for the relationship. That is, while you may be a couple that looks and even acts completely vanilla in most ways, there is always a power exchange being expressed whether it's a hidden or specialized piece of jewelry the submissive (or even both) wears, that the dominant always drives, that the dominant always takes the first bite before the other eats, that the dominant controls the remote, and a myriad other ways that may be subtle or never noticed by others but are things that help maintain the D/s dynamic. If you want to be in a relationship with your dominant beyond strictly a D/s dynamic these sites could prove to be useful.

If you're going to use one of these options it's best to state as near the top of your profile as possible that you're kinky and seeking a relationship with BDSM elements or a D/s dynamic. Also give a quick mention on how you identify, such as being a submissive or switch or bottom or anything else. Since the sites are primarily for the vanilla people, being honest about something like D/s dynamics being important (or even required) for you will help save everyone time and frustration by letting them know immediately without having to scroll all the way through a profile to find out they wasted their time because they're not into kink. One option is to include a link to your profile at another site such as FetLife (see below) so those who are interested in kink as well can find out more about the kinky-you. However, be sure to check the site policy on putting links to other sites as several will not allow it since it means driving traffic away from their own site. Also, remember these are vanilla sites so focus more on your everyday self and interests in your profile and let the kinky details come out through the emails instead.

DO NOT POST NUDES on your vanilla-based profile. While vanilla profiles don't mean sexless, most people who are there do not want to see nudes and it's a surefire way to get yourself skipped over or even blocked so that you don't show up in that person's future searches. Some sites will not allow the posting of nudes at all and to do so could wind up getting your pictures removed, your account limited or suspended, or your profile banned entirely. It's also not advised to do this because of how easy it will be for someone to accidentally come across your profile (see warning below).

Word of Caution: Vanilla dating sites are extremely popular and can be easily accessed by almost anyone. This could put you at risk of having anyone in your life happen across your profile whether they are purposefully looking for it or just happen across it and realize it's you. If you're going to include anything about kink or D/s dynamics in your profile on vanilla pages be aware that this can easily out you.

OkCupid (OKC): They have some blog material about BDSM and do not seem opposed to BDSM seekers/profiles. They were a bit slow to get updated regarding gender identity and still seem a bit behind the eight-ball in that regard. However, given its longevity and popularity, this is a good option to consider.

Plenty of Fish (POF): Unfortunately this site is still very negligent when it comes to the TGNC community and there are even posts about wanting to have the ability to just mass block TGNC people. I've even had my own profile deleted from them without even mentioning kink, just that I was transgender. This site is available, it can be an option, but I would definitely exercise caution and don't be surprised if you find your profile deleted and no response from the admins.

Tinder: This has become an extremely popular app as it requires very little effort to set up or navigate. It does significantly limit how much you can put in your profile so pick your words carefully. Again, be sure to include BDSM or D/s dynamics as being important to you so people can see right off.

An additional word of caution: Be aware that Tinder primarily operates by connecting to your Facebook account. While they've made changes to allow you to just use a phone number (although limiting your feature access), the majority of people use the ease of signing up using their Facebook account and this can wind up providing someone with a massive amount of personal information if they want to dig enough.

Other sites: Zoosk, eHarmony, and Match are all viable and popular options but tend to be less popular or less conducive to those who need BDSM or D/s dynamics as part of their relationship.

Kinky

Alt: This **used** to be the mother of all adult sites that was designed for interacting with members. It, however, is for anyone interested in anything sexual no matter how mild or extreme. It's based purely on sex with little care about anything else. It also is a pay-site with somewhat steep pricing tiers. While it does offer free memberships, the free portions of the site are severely limited. This is a place to go if you're just looking for cyber-sex or sex in general.

Bondage (Bcom): This also **used** to be an amazing site and was specifically designed for those who are into the lifestyle. Best of all, the majority of the site was free with a couple of premium features requiring paid membership but the rates were typically reasonable and the features were worth the few extra dollars. It had incredible features and usability but eventually was bought by Alt and immediately run into the ground. If you weren't being slammed with massive amounts of ads you suddenly found the features you loved being locked away under Alt's pricing scheme.

FetLife: The current **best** site and still holding true. The site was designed in direct response to the Alt takeover of Bcom and, as such, remains almost entirely free with a few premium features needing paid membership, but the membership rates are very reasonable. This site offers a slew of features ranging from groups, unlimited fetish listings, unlimited emailing, unlimited pictures, journaling, ability to mark your pictures and journal entries to be viewable either site-wide or for friends only, and plenty of user-based videos. This is probably the best bet for anyone and even if you use other sites this is definitely one place you want to have an account. While trolls and fakes are everywhere, you tend to get a bit more quality over quantity with this site as it's designed to be a communication hub for kinksters and not necessarily a dating site.

CollarSpace: This used to be CollarMe but underwent a traumatic split and became CollarSpace. Regardless of the name, the general incarnation has been one of quantity over quality. That is, it seems to attract the greatest number of trolls, HNGs, scammers, FinDoms, and the other less-appealing types. It's designed to be more of a dating-type site and while it's completely free and does offer some features the site also boasts significant issues. Random words are often censored so if you type something like "command" it will remove the "com" because that could be construed as a link. It also has managed to remove almost all punctuation from profiles and emails, as well as removed the journal feature access although pre-existing journals remain available but cannot be edited. It is also attempting to individually approve every single profile every time one is created or updated and could take months for that to be approved. If you're willing to tolerate the poor site design and maintenance and understand that site support will never respond to anything you send them, having an account here could be helpful in drumming up some interactions. Just remember, the majority of those interactions will likely be with fakes or those who just want to play online at something spicy with no intention of going to real life.

Recon: This site is dedicated to men seeking men (including trans men) who have interests in a variety of kinks and fetishes. You will find a lot of interest in NSA arrangements, many profiles that are either blank or contain just a few words, and that both the profile and chat options have character limits. While it is a men-seeking-men site, do not assume all are gay because there are a lot of guys there who are interested in other genders or do not care about genders at all but do respect that this is a site with a specific client base. The gay, kink and fetish scene is a unique world unto itself and this site caters to those interests.

Apps/Chatting

While many sites offer a chat, email, or near-live chat/email system there are a plethora of chatting options available outside of those available on a site. Non-site related apps have the benefit of not being recognizable as being kink-related and they offer a good deal of anonymity – which can be a double-edged sword. While it's a good thing to protect yourself and to expect others to be diligent about their privacy it also means, however, that there's nearly no recourse if there's an issue nor is there a way to really verify with whom you're speaking. Some of the apps have become so popular that some sites have discussion boards, threads, and even groups dedicated solely to exchanging your "handles" or "usernames" on the apps for those interested in talking to anyone for any reason, although it's mostly for cyber-sex.

If the app is clearly for sexual purposes odds are you will not be able to find it in app stores, especially after more recent crackdowns. While certain sites have apps for one or more phone operating systems, you may not be able to access them for download anymore. If you have managed to download an app that may be banned or "flushed" from app stores in the future you may not be able to access updates either, although often the core functions of the apps still operate. However, "generic" apps like the "safe vanilla" dating kinds or general chatting apps are often available with no complications since their purpose is not necessarily sex or "deviant" based. Some companies who had or currently have apps that have been deemed "adult" or "inappropriate" are fighting the policies of these app stores but it's an uphill battle so do not be surprised to see apps come and go.

WhatsApp: This is a comprehensive app as it allows users to not just text but to also share videos and pictures and even make calls. This gives many users a good option to chat with strangers and exchange media content or even call without giving away your personal cell number. If you have a great chat going with someone or even if you're experiencing a potential issue and need to save the chats they can easily be backed up to the phone or Google Drive. Just remember, however, that means the "save" feature works both ways so anything you send to someone else can be saved by them as well.

Be aware, however, that this is also a Facebook-owned app and could easily connect to your personal Facebook account, whether you realize it or not. In fact, there was some concern a little while back that WhatsApp was sharing your data with Facebook.

Kik: This is one of the top apps if you want to chat and still be anonymous or at least protect your privacy. Some of the things that make this a great app for protecting yourself are also things that can (and do) be abused by someone with ill-intent. The app doesn't require a phone number to register or associate with your account which is great to protect against someone gaining access to your private number but also means anyone can get an account on the app with no issues. It works on providing secure and allegedly untraceable messaging which, again, can be a double-edged sword. I emphasize "allegedly" untraceable because nothing is 100% foolproof, especially online. The app also allows for sending pictures and videos for those interested.

Viber: While this app also allows for messaging it's primarily intended for calls (including video calls). It's a great option to use to help keep your personal cell number private. A major bonus option to this app is that it allows for international calling free of charge.

Google Voice: This is also a phone call-based service, although it too can provide text message abilities. This typically requires you to input your existing cell phone number and then sign up for a new number (including picking from any area code you want). That new number will then act as a relay directly to your existing number. It has a handy feature of transcribing your voicemails (although it still needs some work on accuracy). It can operate without a standard phone number connected to it, but you may have to remove it after signing up and it does remove some of the features. You can also use this service through their web interface.

Tinder is also an app although since its entire purpose is for dating or hooking up, I opted to include it above under the Vanilla dating options.

Video-Based Chatting:

Chaturbate: This is currently the go-to option for video-based cyber-sex. This is extremely popular because it's live video feed organized into several categories and offers a variety of options. Its primary purpose is to allow cam performers the chance to make money for those performances and can be a mix of porn-star quality performers to your everyday average Joe/Jane. It's currently the most popular adult cam site/app but it's by no means the only option. There's also *LiveJasmin* and *Bongacams* as well as some others that aren't as large-scale.

Certain kink sites will allow you to access a video chat feature and while the overall site may be free to use, video features are often considered a premium feature and require some kind of membership or payment. Since video streaming can be a drain on bandwidth it's not surprising that this is a pay-for-use option but there are several sites that do carry this feature. It can be used as a way to engage in a regular chat room environment, a way to speak one-on-one, and definitely as a way to perform sexually for one or more people. The video chat features built into sites like this are often not used (and sometimes are forbidden from being used) as a means to make money. If you want to perform for money then you should use these other options.

Safety/Privacy Apps

Regardless of what app, site, or service you use there are several things you should use or get in the habit of doing to help protect yourself from online predators, scam artists, and even big companies. These are generally good habits to get into as an Internet user in general, but will also go a long way to helping you avoid potential risks to your privacy when talking to such a wide range of people and within a niche community that, unfortunately, makes it easy for scammers to hide.

Virtual Private Network (VPN): It's highly recommended that anyone, regardless of what you do online, get a VPN service. With the ever-changing policies on privacy, companies using your information without your knowledge, and just general online savviness a VPN is never a bad idea. It's a good idea to read up on several and compare their features but the general core purpose is that a VPN hides your IP and masks it with another, including those from different countries. While it doesn't hide the bandwidth from your ISP it does hide the "what" from them. Not all VPNs are the same so research your options carefully. One feature that several VPNs do offer, however, is "multiple instances" which means you can use it on more than one computer and some even have apps so you can use it on your phone. Be aware, however, that when you use a VPN some websites may not work properly so it may take some trial and error.

Alternative Phone Numbers: As previously mentioned, there are several apps available that give you calling and/or texting abilities. It is strongly recommended that you use an app that provides you with an alternative number, like Google Voice, that you can give out in place of your regular phone number to handle all of your text/calls pertaining to people you've found online.

Alternative Email: It's always advised to get a second email address which you can do with a slew of providers who offer email addresses for free. When signing up for this secondary email address be cautious about what information you provide during the sign-up stage as using your real information can still make the address (and you) traceable. Even if you do use your real information to sign up for the account, immediately go into the settings and explore the "Display Name" option as most of them have this and change it to something other than your real name. Use this email address to sign up for your sites, your apps, and to give out to anyone who wants to chat further. If you use a Gmail account you can then gain access to the Google Hangouts feature which is an Instant Messaging program.

DuckDuckGo: This is a search engine and a good alternative to big ones like Google that track everything you do. Because its sole emphasis is on privacy and not tracking its users, all users will get the same results rather than results being tailored to the user based on all the hidden stuff Google and others track about you. This does mean, however, that sometimes your searches may not be exactly what you want or you may have to scroll past the first page to find just the right link but it does provide a good alternative if you're tired of your personal information being used without your knowledge.

Notification Settings/Contact Listing: It's important to be aware of how you have someone entered into your contacts because that's how texts and other messages may flash across your phone's screen. Additionally, with the way that everything is so interconnected and sites/apps wanting more and more access to everything digital in your life many will import your contacts whether you realize it or not. Secondly, when you receive a notification about email, text, or messages through an app most phones (and apps) are pre-set to show the notifications in your lock screen, home screen, and through a banner notification. These notifications are usually set to show at least some portion of the text/email content to give you a general idea if you want to respond immediately or if it's something that can wait until later. Those notification settings, however, mean that anyone who happens to see your phone might see something they shouldn't, such as if you left your phone on your desk at work just to use the bathroom and a text flashes across the screen that "Mistress/Master Leather Fluff calling you a submissive" or something else naughty that a co-worker/boss happens to see in passing.

Notification settings can be adjusted to just show the name with no preview, you can turn off where the notifications appear such as letting them appear everywhere except the lock screen, or you can remove notification pop-ups entirely and just let the app show you a number indicator on the app to tell you how many messages you have.

Browser Features & Safety

Browsers typically have a good variety of add-ons and some of them are worth exploring to help protect your privacy while other features offer you privacy right off the bat. Some may offer multiple features while others offer only one feature. Some work wonderfully handling a multitude of features while others function only so-so because it's trying to do too much at once so you may be better off with two or three high-performance add-ons that each handle only one task. While there are plenty of good options out there and it may take some trial and error to see what you like the best, I've included a couple that I use (on a Chrome browser) as a jumping off point. Some add-ons may not be available on every browser either so you may have to explore alternatives.

It's important to remember, however, that the more add-ons you include on your browser, especially Chrome, the more "instances" you will find running in the background of your computer. If you're like most people these days you will have a browser window with at least one tab open almost all the time. Every tab may create a new "instance" because that add-on is now working on each and every one of those tabs and this could cause sluggish performance or even browser crashes if you open too many tabs. This will vary by the user based on browser and computer specifications, but it is something to keep in mind.

Additionally, bear in mind that some sites may protest the usage of these privacy protectors because they make money and continue to operate because of the information they can collect from you and your patterns of use. Be careful and read "alerts" carefully that make it seem that you cannot use the page because you have a blocker in place, since oftentimes you can bypass the alert and continue to use the page without relinquishing your privacy. Some sites, however, do force you to disable some blockers in order to view their pages, but I am of a mind that if a site is going to create a hostage situation that requires me to forfeit my privacy I will find the information I want elsewhere, especially considering that it's very likely the same information is available through a variety of other sites. It's entirely up to you on what you want to do with your personal information, but just be aware of what's happening while you surf the web.

Adblock Plus: This add-on provides a variety of settings that allow you to customize how much it blocks, if it will allow certain things to come through, and even allows the user to create their own filters for what is and isn't blocked.

Popup Blocker Pro: This is a very simple add-on that functions well but the only user-feature available is the ability to whitelist a site. Otherwise, the add-on is devoid of features but that doesn't mean it's not effective.

Grammarly: This is not a safety or privacy feature but it's something everyone should have installed if they can use it on their browser. It will catch a significant amount of spelling and grammatical errors across most sites. It doesn't seem to work with some chat-based platforms like Google Hangout web interface. However, it is a fantastic feature to use if you're planning on making journal entries or take part in discussion forums. It will help catch a large portion of errors and help you present in a much better manner to those reading what you post.

WebRTC Network Limiter: If you use a VPN service sometimes "IP Leak" happens regardless of the quality of the VPN service. This means that your real IP address is still visible to some or all of the Internet and that means you can be tracked by someone with even a little Internet savvy. Some VPNs develop special features within their service to counteract IP Leak but it will never hurt to add an extra layer of protection. You can download this (or similar) add-ons to help stop potential leaks.

Incognito/Private Browsing: This is a feature in most, if not all, browsers including those on your phones. This is **not** the same as a VPN as your IP is traceable and your ISP (or others) can still see what you're browsing. What it does, however, is prevent the browser from keeping a history of the pages or date you access so you won't have to constantly clear your browser history. It's advised to use this function if you're looking up porn because browsers now have "autocomplete" or "smart suggestion" features that will pop up a slew of recently seen/typed page suggestions. If you're looking up porn or anything kink related on your regular browser those may appear in the suggestions by mistake and could be awkward if anyone else sees it or uses your phone for anything.

Overall, this should give you some general places to start and, at least, some things to give some serious consideration. I recommend researching things further and definitely exploring what options are best for you as what's available can change overnight. While common sense is very important to avoid being duped by someone online, it's important to realize that some people are well-versed or at least knowledgeable enough about tracking things down on the Internet that it could mean you're unknowingly leaking out private information. While you shouldn't be paranoid to the point where you never want to go online again or are suddenly covering your house in tinfoil, you should be practicing some basic Internet privacy and safety steps. Do not use: "I'm computer illiterate" or similar excuses as a reason not to take some basic steps. If you're genuinely without these skills then seek out a trusted friend to help you or even take classes about basic computer skills at your local library.

Chapter 14

Groups, Message Forums, & Chats

Most sites will have at least one, if not all, of these venues available as they help provide a sense of community and allow for live, instant interaction. However, they're also plagued with those seeking cyber-sex/cyber scening or just a general desire to be obnoxious. With the popularity of social media it's incredibly rare to **not** encounter some kind of Internet troll and, in fact, odds are pretty good you've even seen articles announcing that some celebrity or another has left social media because of the number of abusive trolls. Our lifestyle is no different and so we will, unfortunately, encounter Trolls, HNGs (Horney Net Geeks), or SNERTS (Snot Nose Egotistical Rude Twits) whether we want to or not. These are things to avoid interacting with whenever possible but it's absolutely something you do not ever want to be labeled.

While the Internet is a big place, lifestyle-centric sites are still a pretty niche community so news will travel fast on those who fit any of those above categories. While there's never any real way to know or understand why someone feels inclined to attack people online, it's often done just to instigate and the more you engage with them the more the trolls win and enjoy themselves. If you encounter such a person, regardless of how they claim to identify, just report them to the moderators or site owners, block them, and move on with life. The second you disengage is when the fun for them stops. I can't tell you how many times a troll starts with me in any number of social media or website forums and the second I say, "Ignore the troll <block>," they disappear even though I never actually blocked them. Just the thought that they could be blocked and can no longer engage in their trash talk is enough to shut them down.

Other than the trolls that like to just stir up drama for no reason there's also an alarming amount of catfishing (fake accounts) that are created. For some reason, it seems to be primarily men who will activate accounts as females as either dominant or submissive alike. However, it's not all men who are time-wasters. Many women who are wannabes or who just like the concept of kinky sex but have no idea how to go about it in real life or cannot do anything in real life often find chat rooms or forums to be a way to get off and enjoy their "naughty fun" without actually having to do anything. If you're new to these communication options you will have to learn by trial and error, but the fakes can become more easily spotted as you gain experience. As you navigate the website, you'll eventually learn to focus on the more realistic groups, chats, and forums. Take the tips discussed in previous chapters and apply a dab of common sense to these portals of communication and you should be able to avoid the bulk of these nuisances.

There is nothing wrong with wanting to get a little cyber action. However, you need to take it for what it is – a completely detached, no-strings, masturbation session. If you decide to follow this road it is best to let others do the 'propositioning' rather than trolling for it. If you are not the one actively seeking it out, then you won't develop a reputation as a cyber-sex troll. Just remember, these little "chats" are momentary releases, often talking about things in unrealistic ways, and will almost never develop into a real encounter or a real-life relationship with a dominant.

If you don't want to wait to be propositioned for a little cyber-sex and that's all you really want to spend time on for the moment then be upfront about it in your profile or your messages. Some sites have chat rooms or forums dedicated just for getting a little action going and anyone entering those areas should expect the conversations to be strictly masturbation fodder. Additionally, there's a slew of sites and apps available now that cater to just cyber-sex and especially to keeping yourself anonymous while indulging. This was covered in more detail in the **Tech It Out** chapter.

In addition to learning how to avoid fakes, it's equally important that you acquire the skills to present yourself as respectful, intelligent, and willing. This is truly your time to shine and generate interest, versus sending out emails blindly and praying for a response. When you become active in one or more of these mediums, you begin to get to know some of the regulars and eventually develop "friends" who you can learn a great deal from, but also those who may be able to assist or guide you in finding places, groups, or even specific people, both on and offline, to pursue.

Groups

Communicating within groups can help limit some of the ambiguousness of just sending out random emails then hoping for a response that may never come. You are bound to get some type of interaction, and often fairly quickly, in mediums other than an email exchange. Posts may take a couple of hours, or even days, to generate activity, but more likely you'll begin to get responses within minutes, especially on active sites or groups.

This venue allows you the chance to think about what you're saying and how you're saying it as well as increasing your potential audience. Also, be aware that just because someone hasn't responded doesn't mean they aren't paying attention. This is called "lurking." Lurking can be good practice when you first join a group in order to get a feel for the dynamic, as each group has their own 'flavor,' but don't remain a lurker. The goal here is to establish a (good) reputation online and that can only begin by actually putting yourself and your thoughts out there. Make sure you read the rules for each and every group (and reread them if necessary) before posting but make sure you actually do start posting, whether it is simply in response to others or by generating your own threads.

Don't join every group that seems interesting on the same day and expect to be able to follow all the topics or be able to respond to everything. This is simply too overwhelming and chances are you just won't have the time. Take a moment to explore the groups that are available, find some of the more active ones (don't gauge this solely on how many members are in the group), and read through some of the topics. In many cases, you can typically see at a glance when the last post was made, and if it's been a couple of weeks or more then figure the group isn't that active and you may want to opt out of that one and find another that's more engaging.

Depending on the site design you usually won't have to subscribe/join the group in order to read the discussions, however, in most cases, you will have to join if you intend to respond. If there are ten groups that focus on spanking you don't have to join all ten. Watch the activity for a couple of days or check the time stamps on when the last few posts were made. Find ones that seem to have a posting rate that you feel comfortable with and join just those one or two groups. On some sites, groups can even be specific to a town, state, or region such as the NC Spanking Fetishists (not a real group, just an example). This tells you that the majority of the people in the group live or work in NC (North Carolina) or are in the NC area frequently enough that they felt the group was appropriate for them. It also tells you that these people are specifically interested in the spanking fetish as either giver or receiver (or both). It's likely not the only fetish these people enjoy, but it is one they enjoy to a certain extent that warranted them joining this group. So, if you live in California this specific group might not be the best choice.

While you're perusing the threads in a few of the groups that interest you, ask yourself, "What can I contribute to this discussion?" And, equally important, "What can this group provide for me?" While some groups may have a few posts you find very interesting, is there enough to hold your attention? You can bookmark them for reference, but if you don't plan to truly interact in the group it might be best to skip it or check back occasionally just to see if anything interesting has come up, without clogging your feed with unwanted posts. But if you feel there are some wonderful topics or that the "vibe" of the group seems to be in sync with your own, then by all means join it and jump in on the fun.

Once again, just remember, read the rules if the group has them available. There's no point in getting censored, timed-out, removed, or banned after your first post because of a mistake. Group creators/ moderators who provide rules have done so for a purpose and while some can be incredibly long-winded and repetitious and most of them follow "common sense" basic manners, they were put there for a reason so you should take a moment to read them. One of the most common rules that you will encounter will be those pertaining to posting personal ads. A few groups are designed just for that very purpose while others might have designated areas for ads. Posting ads (even ones you think are cleverly disguised but really aren't) in groups that do not allow them or outside the designated area(s) will often result in them being deleted. It also could result in you being put on the "troll" list with its users by developing a bad reputation or a warning from the moderators. Typically moderators will not remove or ban a user for one mistake, but it's definitely possible and completely up to the moderator's discretion.

In general, these groups are a great way to share ideas, seek help on a subject, ask for resources to learn about something, provide advice on any number of subjects, and generally interact with others around a central theme. There are times when the posts will contain resources and citations or links to something as a reference to back up the post but most of the time the posts are opinions. **A word of caution about opinions** – remember that not everyone will share your opinion and vice versa. Most groups discourage, and will actively prevent, "flames" or attacking of others. If an opinion bothers you, you either need to have the self-control to speak to the moderator if you feel it violates a rule, or simply ignore the post or thread. For some reason, there's a significant trend that people feel compelled to write a response when they disagree with something for no other purpose than to just say how adamantly they disagree. This doesn't add anything to the overall experience and does nothing other than stroke your ego that you've made a statement in some way. Don't say things like: "That's stupid, I can't believe anyone would even think that." Or even things like: "No way, I totally call BS on that." If you do feel inclined to post a disagreement then do so in a productive and "non-flame" manner and act like a reasonable adult. Explain why you don't agree with the post or ask the person if they could expound on their thoughts further because you're having trouble understanding the concept. Overall though, if you're interested in posting just to call out the fact that you don't agree, just save your time and move on to another discussion.

Internet groups are meant to provide an open forum for engaging in dialogue with the chance to learn from alternate views and opinions. You should exercise self-control and broaden your mind. It's very important, especially now more than ever, to realize that you can disagree with someone and not engage; you can disagree with someone and not hate or attack them; and/or you can have an intelligent discourse with someone in such a way that you're exchanging ideas and not forcing your opinions on each other. Most people, especially dominants, do not want close-minded or ignorant people in their life.

At this stage, especially if you're new to the site or the lifestyle, it's best to start slow and easy. You've found some posts that pique your interest and you'd like to get involved. If it appears the topic has been talked to death, indicated by either the number of responses already on the thread or that the last response was made a while back, you don't need to feel compelled to respond. However, if there are subjects you wish to discuss with those in the group you can join knowing there is or will be something for you to say. In fact, you can bring up your own discussion thread if there's something on your mind or something you'd like to ask. First and foremost, you should skim through a couple of pages, within reason, to see if your subject has just been discussed. Generating a brand new thread extremely similar to one posted the day before can result in your thread being closed or moved and does nothing to indicate that you are attentive to detail. Remember, attention to detail is a valuable skill for a submissive to have and is often sought by dominants in some capacity or another.

Group owners don't form groups for lurkers but we understand many enjoy reading without feeling an obligation to post. However, since you're here hoping to find the dominant of your dreams, being a lurker is not advised. Now that you have joined a couple of groups that cater to your specific interests, you'll begin to see posts from dominants who share that interest and this means you're off to a good start. You've narrowed down the hundreds (or thousands or even hundreds of thousands) of dominant profiles to those who specifically enjoy the same thing you do whether it's focused on a kink, a philosophy, or even a hobby. Having a shared interest is integral to starting any type of communication and providing a foundation for a potential relationship. Also, remember that for every dominant who is posting chances are there are just as many not posting but who may be reading your posts and developing a possible interest in speaking to you further. You can easily gain the interest of a dominant with insightful and respectful posts, even those who opt to lurk within the group. If you write both frequently and well then chances are pretty good that you may hear from the dominant saying: "I've read your posts, very interesting…" This could be the important first step needed to establish a connection with the dominant you wish to serve.

I've mentioned before, but cannot emphasize enough, as it is perhaps one of the biggest issues group owners have with members – the importance of reading the rules of the group. If you're unsure if something you want to post could be against or even just not in alignment with the overall theme of the group, simply ask the group owners. Asking a group owner/moderator to help you avoid a potential issue with your post makes everyone's lives a lot easier and chances are they will be happy to let you know if there's anything you need to stay away from doing. This is especially helpful if you feel your post could rile some members, and when members get riled they could threaten to report you or claim you're violating the rules. While you don't necessarily want to make posts that needlessly rile the membership, sometimes it's okay if done appropriately and having the "all-clear" from a moderator saves you a lot of hassle down the road.

Once you understand the Do's and Don'ts feel free to jump into some conversations since they are, essentially, free-for-alls and anyone is welcome to post or respond. Sometimes the "OP" (Original Poster) will target a question to a specific group or subset but even in those instances, others can typically share their thoughts on the subject matter.

Some basic (and common sense) etiquette goes a long way, so here are some good things to keep in mind. Do not hog (or otherwise known as hijacking) a thread! This means taking the subject off topic or posting so often that you're practically the only one talking. If you want to respond to points made by different users try doing it all in one post using @username1: (your response) @username2 (your response) and so forth. By simply placing the @ symbol followed by the username of the person you're responding to, people can follow along and you can answer several people at once without monopolizing the boards by making several posts in a row for each response. While you may see other people bombarding the threads, don't use that as an excuse to do the same. Though there are bound to be a few of those folks around in nearly every group, most people actually find it annoying. This is not to say you cannot make multiple posts, but keep with the flow of the thread.

When you're responding to someone's comments, many boards will allow you to use a "quote" feature so that you can actually include the snippet from the post to which you're responding. Many will appreciate this so they won't have to scroll back up and find it themselves. This is, essentially, good manners. Some boards will require you to use an HTML code to box in the quote such as using: [quote]*what the person said that prompted your response.*[/quote] In other instances it could be just a matter of using an asterisk: *what the person said that prompted your response.* In most cases you will see their quote in some highlighted fashion to illustrate that this was a post from another user followed by your own response in a different stylization. If all else fails and you can't get the hang of the quoting structure for the site you're using then go old-school. Just type in the user's name and copy/paste the snippet to which you're responding as it still identifies the initial poster, what was said, and then follows up with your comment.

Don't ramble. It's difficult at times to say what you mean, especially in posts that talk about feelings/sensations/emotions. These things are very difficult to put into words even by the most esteemed writers so the average person is bound to have problems along the way. Do try to be concise in your posts as they tend to have a greater impact than verbose droning. And remember, stay on topic.

Watch your spelling, grammar, and structure here as well, perhaps even more so. When you're typing quickly, especially on a topic you feel passionately about, it's very easy for words to get garbled. It's important to remember you don't have to hit the send/post button the second you finish typing the last letter. Take a second to skim through the post and ask yourself, "Did I address the topic or contribute in some way to the conversation?" "Did I stay on topic or lose the point?" "Did the words I picked make sense?" Also, remember to use some of the tools available to you that I've mentioned in previous chapters. Once again, if English is not your native language preface your posts (especially if you're new to the group) with a little statement that you're not a native English speaker or that there is a disability of some kind as to why your posts may have errors. As you post more regularly and people become familiar with your style that type of statement won't be necessary.

Watch your tone. As I discussed earlier, it can be difficult for people reading your post to "hear" what you're saying exactly as you meant it. It's very easy for readers to misinterpret what you said, not clearly understand it, misread it, or to interpret it negatively. This shouldn't scare you away from posting, but take a moment to read your own writing and see (hear) how it could be construed by others, especially any dominants who might be reading your post. We all get frustrated and we all can get passionate and excited about specific topics, but it's important to remember everyone is entitled to their opinions.

Here are some tips you may want to utilize to help convey a specific intent or tone. With gifs and emojis, our lives have become a lot easier when trying to express a certain tonality but not every site is designed to accept or use these yet. Emoticons are generally useable across all sites as it's just a matter of using regular text. However, now that emojis have become so integrated as a method of communication some have forgotten about emoticons, but they can be very helpful to help emphasize the tone of your message. As with anything, certain groups or sites might have specific usages so nothing is truly "universal" but these are generally good options with which to start:

- :-) or :) – is a simple smile that you can use in a variety of ways

- :-D or :D – is a big smile denoting that you're extremely happy about something

- ;-) or ;) – is simply a wink and could mean you're being cheeky, whimsical, or even just giving an acknowledgment

- 0:-) or 0:) – is a happy halo usually meaning you're innocent or playing at being innocent

- :-o or :o – is used for "wow" or to otherwise denote surprise or disbelief

By using the < > bracket you are indicating that this is not "speech" but more an indicator of emotion or action. Here are some examples:

- <veg> – Very Evil Grin, usually associated with you being playfully devilish.

- <snark> – usually used to imply that you're being sarcastic or snarky.

- <sarcastic> – this one says it all. If you are using sarcasm it does not always translate well with the plain written word. To avoid misunderstandings or confusion you can pointedly state you're being sarcastic.

- *s* or <s> – typically means smile.

- *g* or <g> – indicates a grin or could alternatively mean to giggle.

- *w* or <w> – to wink.

I don't want this section to become a dictionary of chat-speech or emoticons as you should be using full and complete words when making posts to groups. However, if you want to figure out what someone else may be saying in SMS language (chat/text-speak) you can perform a search for "Chat slang," "emoticons," or "SMS language" and you will hit a treasure trove of information. The point I want to convey here is that using a little indicator to help emphasize or clarify the intent of your post can help prevent a lot of misunderstandings and hard feelings in the long run. Don't be afraid to use indicators but don't let them be your only method of expression.

Moreover, many groups cater to dominants, with submissives as the "secondary members" and will encourage, or outright require, respect to all dominants in the group. These are typically given names such as "Female Dominants and male slaves" so that, just by joining, you know that this group is catering to females who see males as slaves or submissives. As such, it is always good form to speak in a respectful manner to everyone but most especially to dominants. That doesn't mean you have to be a push-over. In fact, you can even ignore someone, but to speak to a dominant with a snotty tone or aggressiveness will have you shunned or at least red flagged.

If you don't like the tone, theme, or expectations of a group don't make posts fighting about it. In fact, that behavior will likely get you "flamed" and/or banned regardless of the group. Speaking of flaming... don't do it, plain and simple… just don't. Reconcile yourself to the fact that idiots are among us, always and everywhere; that you won't always agree with people or even with how the group is operated. You can play into their mentality by responding and getting yourself worked up or you can simply ignore them and give them no more fuel for their fire. If it's a group you have an issue with then you need to remember that you can unsubscribe just as easily as you joined and, in most instances, can make a group of your own. Either way, there's no reason to start or engage in a flame war because regardless of which one of you "started it," both parties could get a warning email from the group owner/moderators, temporarily suspended, removed, or even banned. If you honestly feel that you were attacked (or flamed) take the subject directly to the group owner/moderator. Calmly explain why you feel you were attacked, include the person's username, the link or copy of the offending post, and leave it at that. Do not pester the group owner/moderator as the matter will likely be handled privately with the other person and you will not be privy to the outcome. Otherwise, employ self-control, be the better person, and simply ignore the comments entirely.

Flaming or attacking is certainly no way to a dominant's heart, but illustrating self-restraint and the calm to go with it is highly appealing. Don't think that by ignoring a "challenge" in a group that you are being weak because, on the contrary, you're actually showing yourself to be the opposite. You are proving yourself to be of strong character, reliable, and controlled while the other person is making themselves look bad all on their own.

Also, take into consideration the overall nature or tone of the specific group. Some groups are specifically geared toward outright sarcasm or even poking fun at people. What may appear as attacks between members might actually be how they banter thanks to a long established online friendship, so don't jump to the rescue to defend someone if you don't know the whole situation. Then again, some folks just don't like others and that may show through in the way they interact within the group. Don't get caught up in their drama and let the moderators handle it.

I've lingered on the negatives, so I'd like to touch on some positive things that you should consider. Be intelligent in your responses and, again, don't be afraid to toss in a little wit on occasion when appropriate. Do maintain a certain level of respect for others in the group and perhaps a little extra dash of respect for the dominants.

While they may not be your dominant they:

- Could wind up becoming that or…

- Could wind up recommending you to someone who will be.

- Could wind up being a lurker who has been following your posts who might send you a private message and be "the one…"

- Could wind up being a great general resource for you in the long run.

This doesn't mean that you have to grovel, kiss ass, or even take abuse from dominants but you should enter into a group or topic with some type of humbleness or humility. While some dominants behave in a manner that all submissives are beneath them or need to be talked to in a certain "domly-dom" manner, it doesn't mean that you deserve it or even need to tolerate it unless that's the tone of the group. Enjoy the use of your block feature when available or simply just ignore the person – just remember not to block the group owners/moderators because that could result in automatically being banned from the group.

Chats

Unlike forums and groups, the chat rooms provide instantaneous responses and more often than not the people in them have every intention of responding rather than being a lurker, otherwise, there's very little point in being there. There are bound to be some who lurk, hoping to watch any cyber action, but chances are if they're not responding they are either "AFK" (Away From Keyboard) or in "PMs" (Private Messages). Some chat features may allow the user to put a "busy" or "away" flag/status next to their username. If you decide to ignore that signal and message anyway, then you are bound to get what you deserve.

Generally, you'll find the conversation in chats fast-paced, all over the topic spectrum, very informal, and even a little difficult to follow when a plethora of acronyms start flying across the screen and dozens of different conversations are being held at once, especially when you hit peak hours and the room fills up. It's also the place where you are most likely to encounter fakes, trolls, and those looking only for a quick cyber-sex session.

Depending on the site, you can most likely enter various chats that cater to specific topics such as "Male dom for fem subs." If you happen to be a male submissive seeking a Femdom this clearly isn't the room for you and you could even find yourself being booted from the room. "Booting" or being "kicked" is a special feature that the owner/creator/moderator of the chat room has that can kick you out of the chat room and send you back into the main lobby or central chat room. If you ever find yourself booted or kicked and you feel it was unjustly done you can try to reach out to the chat owner/moderator (they often have a special indicator or extra bold username), but they may never respond and you may never know the reason. Don't be a troll by repeatedly trying to enter the room. If they don't answer you then move along to a different room or start one of your own if the feature is available.

Although popularly done, you want to refrain from posting A/S/L (Age/Sex/Location) in the chat immediately upon entering unless required to do so or if you're specifically asked by someone in the room. Typically you see this often where the cyber-sex-seekers congregate. Pay attention to the groove of the room before blasting out your personal specs. In fact, it's a good idea to hold your tongue for a moment to see what the topic is but a friendly hello is usually welcomed freely. Chat rooms often have fairly limited space to describe the room and rules before entering. Upon registering someone new entering the room a "chatbot" can sometimes automatically generate a "Banner" of further rules and instructions such as:

- No flames allowed.

- Post (or DO NOT post) A/S/L upon entering.

- Men must ask to enter, remove clothes, or any other similar type of "role-play" or "cyber-actions" to instill upon the user on who is the "D" and who is the "s."

- Type <specific keystrokes> to obtain the rules. – If you are offered this option use it immediately and read what it has to say. This will usually be a 'bot' message that displays the text to you in a private message.

- Do not PM any user without first asking permission in the room – this is a common rule and not following it can result in being booted/banned.

Some rooms are intended solely for "RPG," which means they're meant to act as a game or as a venue for people to pretend they're living in an alternate realm, society, or even universe. In this lifestyle, you'll most often find those focused around the fantastical world of Gor. In these rooms, people will script out actions such as "kajira (slave) so-and-so kneels at Master's feet and waits patiently." While entertaining and even a bit enlightening, RPG dedicated rooms are not the ones you want to focus your attention on to help find a dominant as many of those you'll be interacting with are folks who enjoy the Gor books or otherwise like to pretend to be in a kinky, D/s, or M/s situation but don't (or can't) do it in real life.

Now that we're dealing with an environment where you're exposed to rapid typing, spelling and grammar typically go out the window. You must also contend with the fact that your text field is usually limited, fitting only a few characters at a time versus the virtually unlimited space you have in groups and forums. Because of this, many will write in abbreviations or acronyms. Trying to decipher them can be a little tricky at times but if you watch enough and see them used repeatedly and in context it is usually possible to figure out their meanings, but if you need to ask, then ask – just remember though, a quick search online will also provide you with the answer from countless websites dedicated to SMS and Chat language.

Be prepared for PMs, sometimes from the very moment you enter the room and even multiple ones at the same time. While this is commonly a problem that females experience, it is something that happens with regularity even when it's against the room rules. It's especially prevalent in rooms that are typically geared toward cyber-sex only. It's a rarity that you will make any sincere connections in RPG or cyber-sex centric rooms, but sometimes generalized rooms offer you an opportunity to speak to like-minded people and if visited often enough you will start to generate camaraderie and even friendship with other room regulars. It really does depend on the subject/topic of the room as to what type of people you'll attract for conversation. I have made friends on some sites that allowed me to have people to meet up with at the New England Fetish Flea Market events and those with whom I still communicate on other websites or even by phone/texting and have gotten to call friends.

Some rooms are closely moderated and are meant to stay on a specific topic, allowing those in the room a greater chance to have "real" conversations. Once you find a room like this it's best to remember it and return whenever you can. In these types of rooms you'll be able to engage in legitimate conversation and get to know people better and through a different "vibe" than you would in a random or RPG room.

Alternatively, if you're not finding what you want in the chats, many sites will offer you the ability to create a room of your own. In some instances, you may have to be a paying member, while others offer this as a free service. Either way, if you opt to create your own room you now control the atmosphere and can help weed out the cyber-sex-seekers from those with whom you genuinely wish to speak. Further, some will allow you to make the room private or invitation-only to help prevent the unwanted types from strolling in. As you become more acquainted with the chat rooms and develop relationships within them, making a private room becomes a better option so that you're not interrupted by trolls.

Because of the instantaneousness of chatting, you can more quickly discern the players and trolls from the genuine folks and certainly the more you do it the easier it will become to spot them all. Once again, however, you should maintain a certain level of respect, adhere to any rules that are made available, and try to always put your best foot forward because you never know if that "one" person is there that you click with and want to get to know better.

Message Forums

Message Forums are very similar to groups with the small difference of format and design. They are typically viewed as message boards where you can join once and then read all the main and sub-topics in their own sections versus having to join each group individually. Many sites will opt for this approach as the boards are a bit easier to install and require almost no maintenance (other than traditional moderating) from the site owners.

Inside each main topic area, you may find a listing of rules that should be followed for the threads. Before making any post you should read these to make sure you're not stepping on anyone's toes. As with the other two mediums discussed, using respect and tact is always your best recourse no matter the topic.

In General

Remember, regardless of what method you're using, if you truly experience a problem you can always report it to the owner/moderator of that group, chat, or forum. The idea of interacting here is to allow people who share the same interests as you to get to know you. No matter the topic, there are bound to be a plethora of opinions and views and you won't always agree with every one of them, nor will everyone always agree with your points. It's important to respect that, but as you continue to talk in these venues you'll begin to see regulars, learn who they are, and find those who share similar thoughts. This is a great method of bonding with people and has a greater chance of taking messages into a private setting. This is why it's also important to have your profile up-to-par as someone who begins to see your posts more frequently and enjoys them or agrees with them may very well go to your profile to learn a little bit more about you. And who knows what can happen from there...

Chapter 15

Initiating Email Contact

Many potential submissives, especially those new to the scene, would have already sent out a bombardment of emails at this point. Often they don't mean to come off with the attitude of wanton disregard but because they were unaware of what they were doing, the submissives can quickly become discouraged by the tremendous lack of response. In turn, this may make them a bit bitter or lazy and can result in future emails that are clearly written once and then copied/pasted. The thought behind that is: "If I'm not going to get an answer, why waste time writing a personal email?" You're actually creating your own cycle of error and rejection. If you haven't done any (or all) of the steps I've discussed thus far but you have been sending out emails, this is the first problem – you've definitely put the cart before the horse.

Think of it this way. You wouldn't pick up the phone and dial the first number from the phone book and ask them to go out on a date. Just because you're on a kink site doesn't mean you can still "cold call" any dominant and expect to succeed.

At other times it's simply a lazy person who finds the fantasy of submission sexy but has little desire to live it or, more importantly, learn it. In all actuality, the submissive should wait until reaching this point in the book before they even consider sending out emails. That means you should have spent time working on your profile and getting active in public forums before hitting up any dominants in the hopes of getting something going through private messages.

Now that you've gained some experience on the boards/rooms, perhaps even started to make some friends, and hopefully learned how to address and speak to dominants (believe me, we aren't shy and will tell you straight up, especially in our profiles) it's time to start exploring their profiles. I don't mean do a search for every Female or Male, Dominant, people within a certain age range, or those located in specific areas and then send out a mass email to all of them. It doesn't take a special talent for dominants to see that you copied/pasted your message and so they will usually delete it with no response. If you do manage to get a response, chances are it's to call you out on this lazy practice. Groveling after the fact will fall on deaf ears (or blind eyes, as it were).

By all means, do the searches to help narrow it down to those in your area and within your other criteria, but take the time to actually read the individual profiles. Many will state whether they're looking or happily content with their situation as it stands, so you can further whittle it down. While it may seem tedious and time-consuming to read profiles, you would be spending the same amount of time blasting out emails and making a name for yourself as a troll, so you might as well take the better, and likely more effective, approach and take your time to do it right. You can use the multi-tab feature in your web browser to open multiple profiles in a row and start closing down the ones that can be immediately eliminated as not meeting your needs or not being in the market for a submissive.

Bookmark the pages of the few that seem to really catch your eye and then go back for further investigation. Most sites will allow you to see what groups they are a member of, posts they've made, pictures posted, and assorted comments. Although, keep in mind some details or additional information may be available only to "friends." In their written word the dominant may seem like your dream come true but after reading some of their posts or seeing their pictures, you may realize they might be far too strict or a hardcore player (or perhaps too mild) for your liking. Their posts may directly contradict the 'control' they illustrate in their profile. Another feature to consider on the profile, if available, is what events they might be attending. If the website offers this ability it is a good way to see if they are active in the local community. If you're looking for someone who is active locally and you see nothing listed, this may not be the fit for you. Do keep in mind, however, that some people RSVP to events privately or they may not be attending something that week/month because of private reasons, so a lack of event listings is not always a sure indicator that the dominant doesn't participate and it's just something to consider when looking at profiles.

When you found one that seems interesting, it's time to formulate a message to them. This is where you need to shine the brightest and make your email truly pop above the innumerable others they get that are just plain trash. In fact, read through their profile again and even consider jotting down some notes about things that you can specifically reference when writing your message. Did something strike you as really interesting? Did you have a question or would you like clarification on something specific? When a dominant reads things in your message that clearly indicate you've read their profile you are bound to go up a notch and are thus far more likely to get a response.

Before you start typing, be sure to check their profile to see if they have a specific way they prefer to be addressed. Calling a FemDom Ma'am when she explicitly states she prefers Goddess will be an alarm ringing for her that you didn't bother to read her profile and she could stop reading without getting past your first line. Additionally, this holds true if you are messaging a male and call him Daddy because you like that dynamic and yet his profile says he's not interested in it or expressly states he is to be addressed as Sir. If there is no mention in the profile as to form of address then use their screen name – if it says Mistress so-and-so or Miss, Master, Sir, or whatever else – use that term. If all else fails and the screen name itself is ambiguous then use Sir or Ma'am.

In fact, if their title or honorific is unclear, then simply asking in the first line how they would prefer to be addressed shows that you read their profile, you actually paid attention, and you're looking to make sure you do the right thing from the start. Something along the lines of, "Dear Sir/Ma'am: I apologize for the somewhat informal address but as I thoroughly read your profile I was unable to find what honorific you prefer. If you could please inform me what you desire I will be happy to address you as such."

Here's the important part, you want your email to be short and sweet so that it will make her want to respond to find out more about you but, at the same time, be long enough and with enough information, so as not to seem like a fly-by. Extensive emails should not be the first one sent but, instead, should be reserved after establishing a correspondence.

Things to include in your email are any questions that popped into your mind when you read their profile, especially if anything was unclear or something that really caught your interest. This is where taking the notes I mentioned earlier comes in handy. Did you notice the groups they were a member of and/or read any of their posts? Mention the post by saying you really enjoyed their thoughts on the subject of "such-and-such" in the group "this-and-that." This is a bit precarious as you don't want to come off as a creepy stalker, but you do want to let them know that they were of such great interest to you that you really wanted to know more about them. You can word it something like, "I happened to see your post about 'this' and it really piqued my interest." This is especially great if the dominant's post is what drew you to their profile in the first place. Again, do not be afraid – and, in fact, it's strongly encouraged that you specifically reference something in their profile as this will only help them see that you really did take the time to read it and aren't just spamming them.

Absolutely, positively, without a doubt, avoid blasting them with all your desires and things you want. This screams to a dominant that you're a "do-me sub" or a "top from the bottom" type or generally just don't care about submission and just want your kink fulfilled. In fact, all it says is that you're only into them dominating you with no intention of even getting to know them as a person or developing into something together and you're likely better off just visiting a professional. Unless their profile specifically tells you to mention things that you like, it is actually ideal to avoid mentioning anything about your kink wish list in the first email. First, if they're interested they can read your profile to find out about your desires. Second, many will want to know more about you as a human being before delving into kink.

In the case where a dominant's profile tells you to include your kink interests, keep it within their stipulations and try to word it so that it doesn't come off as a demand but rather as you complying with their orders as per their profile. Otherwise, until they specifically ask for these details, a dominant who you're just starting to message doesn't care if you yearn for spanking, flogging, rope bondage, or anything else. This is why the entire previous chapter **Kink/Fetish Lists** was included so don't blow it now that you're ready to get started with your first message attempt. For those who do want to know, you should word your reply similar to the following:

"I read in your profile that you wanted to know some of my interests in kink. I enjoy X, Y, Z, etc. and I'm seeking someone with compatible interests with whom I can grow and explore."

Something like this lets them know that besides actually reading their profile you can follow basic instructions, which is surprisingly not as common as you may think. It lets them know that you have interests (and if you are curious, but have never experienced something, say so) so they can determine if you enjoy similar kinks. It also tells them that you're interested in growing as a submissive within and under their dominance and guidance and aren't stagnant with just wanting to do only a few things.

Take a brief moment to explain a little about yourself including if you're new or your level of experience. Do not copy and paste your profile nor repeat too much of what's in there. Give a little hint of information that will seem appealing to them and they can find the rest in your profile on their own. If they are only looking for an experienced submissive and you have several years of service under your belt then be sure to mention that, but if you're brand new then save everyone time by not messaging them. "Sir/Ma'am, I saw in your profile that you are seeking an experienced submissive. I'd be happy to provide you with my service history and references as I have 'this many' years of experience." If you do have experience then you can mention some of it in the initial email by including how many you've served, if it was live-in or sessions only, and a couple of highlights on what you did for the dominant but don't get carried away.

If you have only served one or two people you don't necessarily have to include why you separated from them, but it is helpful. However, if you've served multiple people you should volunteer what caused the end of service for at least a couple of them as this provides a dominant with a view of your history. Why do it for a larger serving history? Because just seeing a list of multiple dominants that you've served could indicate a pattern – just like someone with a very long resume of going from one job to the next can indicate there's a problem with commitment or following orders.

We've all heard some variation of: "My master/mistress married and didn't want a submissive anymore," or "My master/mistress wanted someone younger," or "My master/mistress died," or "My mistress moved away and I couldn't follow (or they didn't want you to come with them) for whatever reason." While some of these are bound to be true most of them aren't, and this type of "break up" means there's little chance of getting a reference from the previous dominant or could mean the entire story is made-up. If this is the reason(s) for all your splits from service this can be a very big red flag to a dominant and they will automatically think that you're lying about having any service history since none of it can, apparently, be verified. While these things do happen to submissives and can be valid reasons to no longer be in service to someone, you may want to think about how it will be perceived by another person. Perhaps try, "The previous master/mistress and I knew it would only be a short-term arrangement as they were engaged and knew that once they were married they weren't going to keep a submissive full-time. So I got to serve them for six months on a part-time or temporary basis until they got married." It's a spin on the tale that could help soften the "bullshit" factor and appear more genuine, which is exactly what you want if, in fact, this is the truth. Do NOT spin your story for the sake of making yourself sound better. At that point, you're not "spinning," you're actually lying. That means, if you "left" your previous dominant because you weren't happy with the situation and the way you left was just by ghosting them then do not say "you mutually agreed it would just be a short-term arrangement, mostly for training purposes" because that's a lie and it covers up the fact that instead of communicating with the dominant you took a lazy and irresponsible way out of a situation.

Further, when sending the first email you shouldn't list more than two or three past services (and if you do keep it very brief) but you can say: "And I also served others. I don't want to bore you with a lot of information all at once but I'd be happy to share any details if you are interested." This is telling them not only that you are experienced but you're mindful that their time is important and will still be open about sharing your information. Plus, it gives you something to talk about in future emails. When talking about your experience you should never say, "I have experience with 'pain, CBT, restraints, being a sex slave,'" and so forth. You are now venturing into that grocery list of kinks and it comes off as though you're telling the dominant these are things you expect from them. Rather, you should focus on the types of service you performed (key word here is 'service'), whether it was cleaning house, running errands, giving massages, pedicures/manicures, or anything else that you did for your master/mistress. Not what your mistress did to or for you.

One of the exceptions to talking about your kinks is if there is something that you truly cannot live without when being in service to someone. This should be the one thing that's considered a deal breaker or that you'd be utterly miserable and unfulfilled if it was not in your life. Mention this in the first email or pretty early on in communication because if it winds up being something the dominant doesn't engage in that's something you want to find out immediately. Do so respectfully and without a hint of demand, such as: "Sir/Mistress, I do not wish this to come off as a demand of you, but while I am pleased to do and not do things per your interests and commands, there is one thing that I feel is vital to the type of D/s dynamic I hope to achieve and that is…"

Furthermore, it's important to tell them what you found so intriguing about them and this, once more, comes from reading their profile and/or posts. Most people love to hear complimentary things about themselves but don't come off as a sycophant or that the things you like the most are superficial like saying they're so beautiful/handsome. Dig a little deeper into what you find interesting or attractive like finding their eyes alluring or something they wrote really connected with you.

It's also very important to address anything that may be an immediate concern for them. Dominants will often put things in their profile that say: "If you're outside the area I'm not interested," so if you live outside of that area but feel everything else could be a perfect match you will want to address the issue of distance immediately. Explain that you're willing to commute without complaint, that you travel to that area frequently for work even though you don't actually live there, or that you're willing (or are already looking to) relocate to that area. There's a chance that they will still say they aren't interested because they don't want the hassle or time constraints of someone who has to travel to them from too far away, while someone else may be willing to accept that condition especially if you're willing to relocate if things go well down the road.

Many of us get wonderful emails from potential submissives only to find that getting together for a face-to-face is impossible or that the submissive isn't willing to relocate for one reason or another. It makes the entire time spent exchanging emails pointless and an utter waste of time. If you are restricted by location (as in, you're unable to relocate) then do not send messages to someone outside the area you're comfortably willing to travel. Remember, most dominants aren't going to haul their ass out to you, especially in the beginning. If you develop a good relationship with a dominant and have met several times, then they may begin coming to you or meeting halfway, but if you initiate contact with someone who is a few hours away then you need to understand the expectation will be that you will be doing the traveling. There are even occasions when the dominant is looking to relocate rather than having the submissive move, so this is something to look into and is usually mentioned or indicated in some way in their profile. This could be a great arrangement if you're stuck at your location but are willing to travel initially for meetings with the potential of them relocating later if the relationship progresses to that point.

Also, don't be afraid to conclude the email with a statement that even if they are not interested in you, that you'd still like to be "friends" and be able to talk on occasion, or perhaps see each other in the forums/chats. This tells the dominant you are not putting expectations or ultimatums on them by saying, "If I can't be your submissive then I don't want to bother with you at all." While that mentality is technically okay, it's also burning potential bridges. That person could wind up becoming a great friend, they could wind up introducing you to the local community, helping you by answering some questions or even helping to fine-tune your searches by letting you know what's right/wrong about your approach, or they could even wind up introducing you to the person who does wind up being the best match for you.

You may be surprised that working towards a friendship will result in them wanting to meet up with you as many feel that having a foundation outside of strictly being D/s is important for the dynamic to last and thrive. We have received some great emails but, for whatever reason, the connection couldn't be made and we receive the, "Well, I'd love to still be friends," follow-up statement but then the submissive disappears entirely. You should still touch base and, actually, attempt to maintain a friendship and, besides, you never know if things in your (or their) life will change or if through the friendship you kindle something more and just needed time to spark that connection.

As I have briefly mentioned in a previous chapter, providing contacts or references can be a wonderful leg-up against the competition. If you have people who know you in the lifestyle via munches, groups, events, or past service and you're able to provide them as references, you will certainly gain a better chance at receiving a response than most others. Informing the dominant that you have references and are willing to share them helps instill a little bit of trust and shows that you have nothing to hide. Of course, make sure that you get permission from your references first, before giving out links to their profiles or, worse, their private information.

I cannot express strongly enough the sheer importance of ensuring that you use spellcheck while writing your emails. While your profile should be relatively free of errors, your email should be pristine. Read it, re-read it, and then read it again aloud. Reading something in your head versus reading something aloud or having a text reader app/program read it are completely different experiences. Your mind will automatically self-correct or you will "hear" it how you wrote it when reading silently, but the second you start to read it out loud you will hear the difference and find that it may not be exactly what you meant. If a dominant has to stumble over your email, decipher it, or at any point in time scratches their head wondering what you were trying to say there's a good chance they'll just delete it and move on to the next message. It is okay to use "impressive" words if you do it without sounding like a pompous know-it-all, but for the most part you want to convey your immediate thoughts and interest in a straightforward, understandable, and readable format. It's a sad fact, but most people will be happy to just receive a message that's more than a one-liner and has fairly decent spelling. If your message has substance to it and is error-free you are already a notch above the rest so don't go into overkill territory by using vocabulary that is above-and-beyond, especially if you don't normally use these words in your daily life. If you, however, are a logophile and utilizing sesquipedalian words is commonplace then, by all means, indulge. Just, once more, be aware that it could come off as pompous and while you shouldn't trivialize your intelligence, be cognizant of how it may come across to the reader.

Once again, if English is not your primary language or there is a disability of some kind that prohibits you from writing clearly it is important – most especially when sending an email above all other areas – to state this right at the very top of your message. Otherwise, you will be seen in a negative light and wind up with one more deleted and unanswered email.

All this seems like a lot of work just for one email, but it's vital to remember that dominants get bombarded with emails so you need to do something to stand out from the rest. Besides, remember that as a submissive seeking to serve a dominant a good deal of your life could be service-based, and if putting in a little effort now is an issue then that mentality might lead to bigger problems down the road. You need to ask yourself: "Do I want to waste my time and make enemies or a bad name for myself?" or "Do I want to spend the same amount of time and put my best face forward and stand a much greater chance of success?"

This is a numbers game – there seems to be far more submissives than there are dominants, so the odds are stacked against you from the start. For every genuine submissive there are a plethora of fake or do-me submissives flooding the dominant's inbox. A little extra work, a little extra polish, will tend to get through the muck. Even if you receive a response saying, "I really liked your email but right now I'm not sure if we're a match," or "I'm not looking for a submissive," you can consider that a win. Why? Well, clearly your message wasn't deleted so you did something right to warrant a response. That's far more than many others get, so count it as a bonus and that you're on the right track and not as a discouragement.

Don't think that we don't talk to each other about some of the emails we get, especially those special few who really were off the wall. In fact, there is even a group that reposts those "special" emails so we can all get a hearty chuckle over them. Your goal is to make sure your email never winds up posted to a group like that and ridiculed among us. In fact, we have even discussed some of those special emails at munches and other events, especially if it's someone targeting dominants within a certain area. We talk. Make sure when we talk, that it's not about you.

SECTION THREE:
OFFLINE/REAL LIFE COMMUNITY

The best way to make a dream come true is to wake up.

In other words, put the computer away and

get yourself out there for some real interactions.

Chapter 16

Want to Know
the Secret Handshake?

What's the secret knock sequence to get into the hidden dungeon? How do you know when to give the person walking by you on the street that knowing smirk or a nod in silent acknowledgment of mutual kinkiness? What's the secret password?

While there isn't necessarily a special handshake or secret password dedicated to the lifestyle, there are, however, a variety of symbols, emblems, flags, and specialty codes that the general vanilla public is unaware of, even if they've seen the images before. Seeing these images is not an invitation to announce it out loud, as many who don or utilize any of the codes listed below will still want privacy, but it will give you the knowledge to spot some of "us" among the masses and give that 'knowing wink.'

**Just remember the warning above
in Chapter 3 about outing people**.

Right vs. Left: It's important to understand this first before we get into the actual symbols and codes themselves. This was originally developed in conjunction with the *Hanky Code* (discussed below) that was used heavily in the 1970s. There needed to be a way to determine who was the 'Top' and who was the 'bottom' or, in other words, who was going to 'give' and who was going to 'receive,' respectively.

As a result, the **Left Side** has come to indicate the Top, Dominant, or Giver while the **Right Side** reflects the Bottom, Submissive, or Receiver. When you see the *Emblem* (see below), the *Hanky Code*, or other symbols, you can typically determine how they identify based upon which side the symbol is displayed. While this is a fairly standard cue it is not universal so there are bound to be some variations.

One such variation is the Gorean 'kef' or slave mark. For some reason, this mark is supposed to be placed on the left side of the slave. There is speculation here that when John Norman was writing his books the hanky code was relatively underground and primarily used within the gay leather men's culture, a group Norman likely wasn't overly aware of at the time, which would explain why it's not in sync with the overall symbolism the community uses. The left/right side has since been incorporated into the kink community at-large while the Gorean kef remains to the left. Since it's a fairly easy mark to identify by those in the know it's easy for the community at-large to understand that the kef itself means the person is a slave/submissive regardless of which side it appears.

The Collar: While the lifestyle fully embraces the collar, many will not or cannot wear a traditional black, leather collar in public. Often a collared submissive/slave will have a piece of jewelry, such as necklace, bracelet, anklet or other similar item that's subtle. Certain high-profile jewelry companies make beautiful pieces that include locks, keys, and other symbols that the lifestyle enjoys and have adapted for the subtlety they convey. The submissive can be collared in public without anyone ever realizing it.

While some, often just a very select few, will wear a leather collar in public, this accessory has been taken over by those going for a gothic-look so one cannot always assume Collar = submissive/slave. Additionally, while porn videos and images have a tendency to show Dominatrices in a collar, sometimes even a posture collar (which is very thick and leaves almost no room for moving one's head), in reality, most FemDoms will never actually wear one and, if anything, may don a decorative choker if it goes with their outfit. Do not confuse the porn-image of a FemDom with reality. Some people have used dog tags (both military style and pet tag styles) with sweet engravings etched into them that typically cannot be read unless you look very closely.

BDSM Emblem (BDSMblem Project): As the Internet hit a boom in the 1990s the BDSM community moved online and sought an image in which to help identify itself. One user, Quagmyr, designed and developed the original Emblem (see image below), which has gone on to have tremendous variation in color scheme and design in general, but the core element has remained the same and has become an easily recognizable symbol to the community.

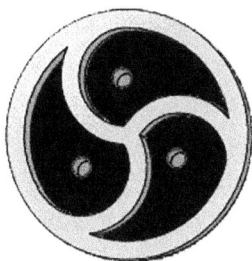

Copyright 1995, 1997
by Quagmyr@aol.com,
used with permission.

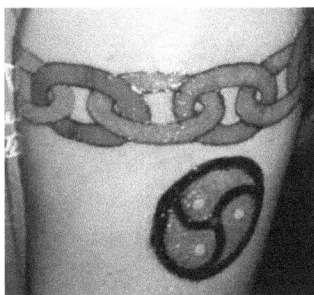

Sir Jude's tattoo

As you can see on the far right image of my own tattoo, it is the same core design but the color scheme was changed to include the colors of the *BDSM Pride Flag* (discussed below). The original design was inspired by a design in the book *The Story of O* by Pauline Réage that, in itself, was based upon the Celtic Triskele. In fact, this has allowed many who wear the Emblem a bit of cover-up, as one can simply say it's based on a Celtic symbol if a vanilla person inquires about the image and the wearer doesn't want to out themselves.

The Emblem itself has many layers of meaning and, as Quagmyr wrote:

"The three divisions represent the various threesomes of BDSM. First of all, the three divisions of BDSM itself: B&D, D&S, and S&M. Secondly, the three-way creed of

BDSM *behavior: Safe, Sane, and Consensual. Thirdly, the three divisions of our community: Tops, Bottoms, and Switches.*

It is this third symbolism that gives meaning to the holes in each unit. Since BDSM *is at the very least a play style and at its greatest a love style, the holes represent the incompleteness of any individual within the* BDSM *context. However "together" and "whole" individuals may be, there remains a void within them that can only be filled by a complimentary [sic] other.* BDSM *cannot be done alone.*

The resemblance to a three-way variation on the Yin-Yang symbol is not accidental. As the curved outline of Yin and Yang represent the hazy border between where one ends and the other begins, so do the curved borders here represent the indistinct divisions between B&D, D&S, and S&M.

The metal and metallic color of the medallion represents the chains or irons of BDSM *servitude/ownership. The three inner fields are black, representing a celebration of the controlled dark side of* BDSM *sexuality.*

The curved lines themselves can be seen as a stylized depiction of a lash as it swings, or even an arm in motion to deliver an erotic spanking. The all-embracing circle, of course, represents the overlying unity of it all and the oneness of a community that protects its own." (Copyright 1995-2013 by Quagmyr@aol.com, used with permission.)

Hanky Code: This is also called "flagging" since you usually wear a bandana which hangs like a flag and it flags others in the know. No one has stepped forward to claim credit for specifically creating the code but it was predominantly used in the 1970s among the Leather Men or gay male population in clubs who were looking for casual sex (remember, this was prior to AIDS/HIV) to help determine who was into what so that they could be more easily approached.

Over the decades, the code has grown to be quite extensive and has since been incorporated within the BDSM community. Given the sheer size and complexity of the code, we won't go into the entire list here but a simple online search for "Hanky Code" or "BDSM Hanky Code" will be sure to give you plenty of reading material if you're interested in the complete list. The BDSM community has adapted the code from its original use. The two share history and similarities but if you specifically search for the "BDSM Hanky Code" you will find versions that are appropriate to our subject. For the sake of staying within of our topic relating to kink, I will list a few examples here as they pertain to the lifestyle. For switches, they can wear the "flag" on either side depending on what they want to give/receive or even put the flag in the middle such as tying it around the belt or belt loop.

Color	Wears on Left	Wears on Right
Black	SM top	SM bottom
Grey	Bondage Top	Bondage Bottom
Blue/Teal	Gives CBT	Receives CBT
Yellow	Likes to Pee On	Likes to be Peed on
Coral	Wants toes sucked	Likes to suck toes
Fuchsia	Gives Spankings	Receives Spankings

As we get into symbols and flags I want to take a moment to give a brief disclaimer. These can all have variations to them. I'm providing just the most common symbols or flags because to include every possible variation would be far beyond the scope of this book. If you encounter a symbol or flag that you're unsure of just ask someone and odds are they will be happy to let you know all about what it represents. If you do not see a symbol or flag here that represents something for you just know there likely is something out there so a quick search for BDSM, Sexuality, or Gender Symbols/Flags will yield an entire world of information.

Symbols: Symbols are used in all aspects of our lives but I wanted to briefly cover a few that you may encounter within the lifestyle, especially since so many in the lifestyle are of such diverse genders and sexualities.

	BISEXUAL: There are several variations on the bisexual symbols to help illustrate specific aspects like if it's male, male, female or female, female, male, but this is a more encompassing symbol to use for bisexuality in general. Public Domain image courtesy of Wikipedia.
	LESBIAN: This is simply the two Venus symbols interlocking. Again, there are plenty of variations on design and color schemes. Public Domain image courtesy of Wikipedia.
	HETEROSEXUAL: The simple Mars and Venus symbols that are most commonly used to denote male and female respectively. Public Domain image courtesy of Wikipedia.
	LABRYS: As discussed under the lesbian flag this symbol can often be used by itself and is used within the lesbian community. Public Domain image courtesy of Wikipedia.

	GAY: Interlocking Mars symbols for indicating gay men. Public Domain image courtesy of Wikipedia.
	PANSEXUAL: Pansexuality is a newer term but has gained a lot of traction. This is typically a step beyond bisexuality as the person is interested in both male and female persons, but it includes those who may identify anywhere within the TGNC spectrum as well. Public Domain image courtesy of Wikipedia.
	POLYAMORY: This symbol is used for those who engage in having relationships with more than one person. As mentioned, this is a complex relationship to which many books have been dedicated. Public Domain image courtesy of Wikipedia.
	TRANSGENDER: There are variations of this symbol and other trans-related symbols that are more specific to indicate Male-to-Female or Female-to-Male. This, however, is the typical "umbrella" symbol for the community. Public Domain image courtesy of Wikipedia.

Flags: Flags have long since been a symbol of reflecting pride and unity. They have been used to stake claims, whether to establish oneself as a part of a group/unified community or to establish land-rights within countries. Flags have developed many meanings and often have their own symbolism worked into the fabric, and the BDSM culture is no different. Over the years many flags have emerged to reflect the various interests and sub-groups throughout the community – there are many choices available. Some flags have been around long enough to become highly identifiable to the general public while others might be known only within their subset.

As with other symbols and codes, the flags have also evolved. For example, the LGBT+ flag (also referred to as the pride flag or the rainbow flag) can sometimes, for example, have a Male or Female symbol inside of it to denote specifically Gay-pride or Lesbian-pride. Once again, it is recommended that you use an online search for "Pride Flags" or "BDSM Flags" to learn about the variations or the history of their development (as some of them have very interesting backgrounds). You will find sites that will show you about all or most of the other sub-groups, including clarification on any of the gender symbols. (Links for the sources are provided in the resource section).

LGBT Pride: The "Rainbow" flag is among those most easily and universally recognized whether you're straight or anywhere within the LGBT+ spectrum. In fact, the Museum of Modern Art ranked the rainbow flag as an internationally important symbol in 2015. It was created in 1978 by Gilbert Baker (sometimes known affectionately as Busty Ross) who sadly passed on March 31, 2017. The colors were specifically selected in the original version which consisted of Hot Pink = Sex, Red = Life, Orange = Healing, Yellow = Sunlight, Green = Nature, Turquoise = Magic/Art, Indigo = Serenity, and Violet = Spirit. Over the years due to various reasons both the Hot Pink and the Turquoise were removed and the "Commercial Version" is what is now most well-known.

Design Variation: To help depict a specific sexuality it is common to see the Venus, Mars, or Bisexual symbols overtop the Rainbow background.

Bisexual Pride: This flag may not be as well-known at large but is definitely recognizable within the LGBT+ communities. It was designed by Michael Page in 1998. While many would immediately assume that the pink triangle represents female and the blue represents male and the purple would be the logical blending of the two this is, in fact, not the case. As the pink triangle was used during WWII to mark anyone who loved or was with someone of the same sex for Hitler's concentration camps, it was reclaimed by the LGBT+ community to be a symbol of power and pride for those who loved others of the same sex. The blue represents those who love those of the opposite sex and the purple is the blending of the two to represent those who love people of either gender.

Bear Pride: While working on a project for his degree, Craig Byrnes set out to develop a flag to represent the Bear subculture that developed amongst gay men. The final version was the design of one of those helping on the project, Paul Witzkoske. The colors of dark brown, orange/rust, golden yellow, tan, white, gray, and black were picked because those were commonly seen as colors of fur of the various animal bears in nature and the black bear paw stamp in the upper left corner is an obvious choice. As one would imagine, a Bear is typically a gay man who is rather hairy. Within this culture there are other identifiers such as Cubs and Otters.

Lesbian Pride: There are a few designs and symbols that have emerged since the 1970s to represent lesbians, although there still seems to be debate about if there is an "official" flag.

Design 1: While the Pink Triangle was used to mark homosexual men for Hitler's camps, a Black Triangle was used to mark lesbians (and any other woman who was considered "asocial"). Lesbians have reclaimed the Black Triangle for themselves and this could be seen most often on a solid background of lavender.

Design 2: The Labrys (see above) was introduced as a symbol for lesbians and can be seen either by itself or being centered over the Black Triangle on the Lavender flag.

Design 3: This flag consists of seven horizontal bars starting with a dark pink through to light pink to white then back up through to a dark red. This flag also sometimes includes a lipstick kiss mark in the top left corner. This is most commonly known as the Lipstick Lesbian flag.

Design 4: The standard Rainbow flag with interlocking Venus (female) symbols.

Transgender Pride: As with so many of these symbols and flags there are variations, although the one (and associated color scheme) that's most widely used was created by Monica Helms in 1999. Helms specifically chose the colors of pink and blue because they were colors traditionally associated with the binary boy/girl. She then opted to use white to denote those who are intersex or have opted to not identify any gender and its position was chosen to help illustrate those in-between. The flag was also specifically designed so that there is no wrong way to fly it as it maintains its scheme either way.

Leather Pride: The flag was designed in 1989 by the late Tony DeBlase and is meant to represent the leather community primarily, but it is sometimes mistakenly used as a representation of the kink community in general. While DeBlase made the flag which consisted of nine stripes that alternated between black and blue with a middle stripe of white, he never made a definitive statement as to the significance of the stripes. Additionally, the flag contains a red heart on the upper left corner and, once again, DeBlase has left it up to individuals to interpret the design elements however they want.

BDSM Pride: This is, technically, a variation of the Leather Pride flag as the horizontal stripes are those of the Leather Pride flag with the variation of the BDSM Emblem being on the flag (often in the center) denoting it as being BDSM Pride. While DeBlase leaves the interpretation of the color scheme up to the Leather community to determine, it's often interpreted as being "black and blue" (like a bruise) for the BDSM community.

Master/slave Pride: The flag was designed by Master Tallen in 2005, and while it's a simple design it stands out clearly. The flag is a solid black background with a solid red vertical stripe that goes almost top to bottom. This stripe is set to represent the Master or mastery/dominance/power in general. There are three thicker but shorter horizontal stripes to the right and centered which indicate lying down in supplication. This is specifically used for a subculture of the BDSM community that explicitly engage in Master/slave dynamics.

Other Flags: There are flags that represent those interested in Adult Baby/Diaper Lovers (ABDL), those into Pet-Play in general, those who are Pups, those interested in Pony-Play, those into Military/Uniforms, those interested in Rubber, and the possibilities go on. Some will take an existing flag and put a symbol over it to help indicate a specific interest (like the BDSM emblem over the Leather Pride colors), while others may be of their own design. Check the links in the resources section if you want to explore what some of these other flags could entail and the interesting histories around their creation.

Once you consider the lingo/terminology, Hanky Code, Flags, Emblems, and even the importance of which side something is on, one can begin to see that we are a vast, developed, and still growing community. While I'm sad to say there is no actual secret handshake, there are many subtle things we, as a community, have incorporated through the years to help signal to others in the know without necessarily, or needlessly, outing ourselves in the process.

Just remember, as is the case with anything in this lifestyle, there is never a clear-cut, end-all-be-all signal or definition. Each group or even each individual will undoubtedly throw their personal spin on things and as the community itself grows new variations and interpretations develop all the time. The symbols and codes illustrated here are brief mentions to simply provide you with a basic groundwork of understanding of what's out there. If you're truly interested in the numerous variations or if you're trying to find what niche(s) you fit into, please utilize the best tool in your arsenal – Internet searches.

Chapter 17

Get Out There!
Munches and Events

As I spent a good deal of time within the North Carolina area, I will be using local NC groups as examples (with their permission) since I have personal knowledge of them. If you're near North Carolina and/or like to travel, some of these groups and events are absolutely worth checking out. However, if you're further away the examples provided can at least give you a general idea of what to look for in your own area or perhaps what to start on your own if one doesn't currently exist in your area.

Munches

These are wonderful opportunities to meet people in a very relaxed atmosphere that never has play happening. The entire purpose is to eat, drink, and be merry with like-minded folks as though you were meeting up with your vanilla friends at a public restaurant. Sometimes the group leaders will have a specific topic for discussion, but in most cases it's a free-for-all and people will talk to all in attendance or hold conversations with a couple of people; there are no rules in this regard.

Most of these groups do not charge any door or membership fees, though if you order anything from the menu you will be responsible for your purchases plus tax and tip. As such, unless you're going to a bar, most often you won't be asked for your ID so these munches are a great way to interact and maintain the utmost anonymity. Most towns/cities have at least one munch but if you're concerned about someone seeing you at a local hot-spot that's being used near your home, you can probably find a munch in a nearby town just as easily where the chances of running into someone you know are less. However, should it happen that someone recognizes you, there is minimal risk involved since munches are very vanilla appearing and if you said something like, "It's a new book club I wanted to check out," no one would bat an eye and it's even possible that the munch may use a vanilla sounding name when placing their reservations that you can easily use as cover.

Usually, munches are held once a month and on the same set day – for example the first Sunday of each month. Occasionally some munches located in larger cities might also host several events throughout the month or may change the location for their monthly meeting to different locations to allow those in different parts of the area to attend without always having to travel.

If you're on a site and found out about the group there, then chances are they will announce when and where the next meeting will be somewhere on that site. Sometimes around the holiday seasons dates will change or be canceled to accommodate other obligations or simply because too few people attend to meet the minimum requirements for reservations. If the munch falls just right with an upcoming holiday the munch might host a theme meeting geared towards that specific holiday.

FOR EXAMPLE:

If you usually go to a small Irish pub in town you may find yourself at a BBQ Joint if your meeting is near July 4th, Memorial Day, or Labor Day. If you normally meet at a Mexican restaurant then on St. Paddy's day you may wind up meeting at the Irish pub.

Changing venues does not happen too often as many places have a hard time accommodating such large groups and once a relationship is established between the restaurant and group, things run a lot smoother than jumping from place to place. However, some groups develop great working relationships with a few restaurants within various geographical areas so that, while they may 'rotate' locations, they are still at the same venue each time it is rotated to that area.

Lastly, there are no requirements on your time for any munches. If you can attend just one, a couple here and there, or every single one it doesn't matter – it's all fine. If you come late, early, or can only stay for part of the meeting that's typically fine as well since it's a very relaxed social gathering. Just don't cause a raucous when you enter or exit. This is one of the easiest methods anyone new to the scene, the area, or new to getting out there locally can embrace. Once you are in your local scene, your chances of meeting a dominant increase exponentially and taking it nice and easy through munches is a great way to get started.

Triangle Munch Group (TMG)

Website: http://www.trianglemunchgroup.org/

Fetlife Group: https://fetlife.com/groups/2943

Not only do I personally love this group and the folks who organize it, but I find it also helps illustrate the absolute awesomeness of munches in general.

First, the group itself is dedicated to educating the community and, as such, they host a fairly extensive (and free to regular members/attendees) library of books covering the entire spectrum of BDSM and the lifestyle in general. Additionally, they host "Tuesday Topical" munches each month. Some topics included:

- I Screwed Up – Now What? How to Deal with "Oops!"

- Labeling Language – What Labels Give Us and What They Take Away.

- How to Deal with Douchebags and Trolls Online or at a Party. Plus, Scene Etiquette and Net Etiquette.

- Bringing Leather to the Community.

- Age-Play for Bigs and Littles.

- Favorite Places to Buy Toys/Gear from the Street to the Net.

As you can see, topics vary significantly and there will occasionally be specific presenters to address some of the subjects, which is how I met Lee Harrington. In most cases, these Topicals are a great open forum where folks can contribute their own thoughts, experiences, insights, and opinions. It was through one of these very Topicals that I learned key verbiage and things to help guide me on my path learning that I was transgender.

This group is also a key example of what I mean by a floating or rotating munch. TMG hosts several munches throughout the month in both the Raleigh and Durham areas. In many cases, the organizers reserve a private room in the restaurants to allow for open discussion on any topic without being overheard by the vanilla patrons. Given the frequency of visits and established relationship the group has developed over time, many of the staff members will work with the group and often have become comfortable enough to overhear some of the conversations without so much as a flinch or batting of an eye. Because the relationship has been so amazingly developed, many of the venues do not charge an automatic gratuity, so it's imperative that you understand how important it is to respect the servers and tip them. They work extremely hard for such large groups, do not judge us, and do not apply a gratuity that many others would, so show respect and gratitude and TIP! TIP! TIP!

Furthermore, TMG doesn't just stop at munches. Oh no, they like to share their awesomeness in even more fun ways. They host a Fashion Show which showcases several categories in which people can compete in various types of fetish attire. They also host an annual picnic for members to gather together for a little BBQ, some (vanilla) fun, and occasionally guest speakers.

If you're in the area, this is one of *the* groups I recommend to everyone just getting involved in the community. It's friendly, accepting, non-judgmental, extremely active, available to any adult, and one of the best ways to make new friends. They also provide announcements for all the other groups and events in the area so this is a fantastic way to learn about everything else going on in the area and book up your calendar.

"Public" Parties/Events

While they might be called "public" parties they are, in no way, open to the general public. It simply indicates that the events are typically an open invitation so you don't have to be a member of any specific group. There is generally an admission fee that could range from $5.00 to $15.00 (although prices do vary) depending on the event, venue, and intent of the group. Events such as these often revolve around playing or scening but can sometimes be educational, such as a class, demo, or practice – or a combination of demo/class and play to follow.

Be aware when attending a party that just because there is play going on, you don't have to play if you're not comfortable. Some couples love public playing and fully embrace it, others love to watch, and others might be without a play partner or have no intention of playing but go to socialize with their friends and make new ones.

It's a wonderful opportunity for you to mingle in a more "party-like" atmosphere and see different forms of play, different styles, and different reactions. You might see things that are new to you and might like to explore... or even things you discover to be a big turn off. It's important to remember there are a million different ways to scene and many ranges of intensity, so try not to let one style turn you off to the concept in general.

FOR EXAMPLE:

You may see a flogging scene with an extra heavy (such as latigo leather) flogger where it appears the dominant is hitting very hard as the heavier leather can cause a deep "thud" sound. However, upon watching the scene you may be interested to learn what it feels like or perhaps determine you're interested in something a little lighter.

Generally, those who are in a scene are well aware of how they like to play, the intensity they are comfortable with, and their limits but just in case a "DM" (dungeon monitor) will check in on the situation or be nearby to ensure things remain safe. Rather than focus on policing or judging a scene, you should view the situation as, "Hmm, that flogging seems interesting. I might like to try that but a bit lighter." As a side note for those very new to the scene and the implements used – floggers (and other tools) come in an extremely wide variety of sizes, designs, and materials with each one designed to deliver varying sensations from soft and sensual to hard impact or stinging. This is a good time to even begin to notice how submissives enter sub-space, their expressions, and their reactions. Watch how the dominant performs and note how and where they're hitting and where the submissive seems most responsive. Everyone reacts differently ranging from almost no reaction to crying to moaning in ecstasy to flailing around like crazy. Try not to let yourself be alarmed by the variations as, again, the players are often couples who know well the reactions they will get and in many cases will actively seek to obtain that reaction.

Alternately, you might just as easily see an extremely light flogging and think, "Geez, what's the point? You can barely feel that." This is usually considered 'sensation play' or might be the submissive's first time being flogged and the dominant is going slow as they explore the new sensations. It's important not to give quick judgments about the scenes or the tools being used and try to just enjoy what's being displayed. Take from these scenes as learning experiences and learn about possible things you might want to explore and, as you grow through experience, can begin to gauge what types of tools and intensities you like best.

A public party, especially a play-based one, can seem overwhelming but keep in mind three very important things:

- The people playing have negotiated the scene, DMs are there, and the play is "SSC" (safe, sane, and consensual).

- No one is expecting you to play, nor will force you to play.

- You are never forced to watch something and are free to move about the space. There are often different zones/areas at such events so if there's a scene going on that you're not interested in you can always move to a different zone.

Just because you identify as a submissive doesn't mean you don't have a voice. You are **ALWAYS** free to politely decline an invitation to play, but if you should ever feel pressured or just aren't sure how to handle a proposition, speak to a DM or the organizers and they'll help handle the situation. These events are designed to be fun and exciting, and many of the organizers and DMs are there to ensure everyone is having a good and safe time and to help you get the most out of the experience so don't be afraid to seek out event staff. However, never interrupt a DM who is monitoring a scene – always seek out someone who is not actively monitoring unless it's an emergency. DMs and organizers will often wear accessories (like a certain color glow stick) or specific clothes (such as a shirt that says Event Staff) that will make them stand out.

This is an optimal experience when you can see someone you may be interested in and watch how they play, how they interact with others, and importantly, how others interact and respond to them. Say, for example, that you've spoken with someone online or through other events and they seem to always say the right things but now you see there's a very cool response to this dominant by other attendees at an event. It could be a cue to investigate further before committing to this person. Has the dominant said that they attend a lot of events and is very active in the community, but you see virtually no one knows who they are at an event or they aren't talking to anyone? It could be an indication that they are not being completely honest with you.

Alternatively, be aware that popularity does not equate to being a good dominant. Knowing how to chat and schmooze with people is completely different from knowing how to use the tools of our lifestyle effectively and safely. Watch as the dominant plays, what they like to do, and how well they handle aftercare. Watch to see if they are hitting the target areas, paying attention to the submissive and scene and **not** the crowd around them (performing for the crowd/attention and not paying attention to what they're actually doing), and if they take care of the submissive afterward. Remember, just to play a little bit of devil's advocate, not all dominants do aftercare nor does every scene warrant it and you may not know what they've discussed and agreed to beforehand. If the dominant abandoned a submissive who needed aftercare you will typically hear whispers go through the rumor mill so you may want to exercise caution but remember, while rumors can hold truth they often don't consider the entire story.

Once again, while it may seem overwhelming, try not to be uptight. It's a bit more difficult to talk in these settings as there's usually music and/or a lot of people, but smiling (without looking crazed or like a Cheshire cat) and keeping your body language open will entice people to come up to you. There is often a designated social area where you can mingle and talk openly. While I will discuss basic etiquette at parties briefly, always remember – do not interrupt a scene and that includes talking in a disruptive manner during one.

Eventually, you will begin to meet a few people through groups online and off and/or at munches so the more things you attend the more you'll begin to expand your networking base. This is how you'll begin to have the best chance at meeting someone you may be able to connect with.

For the groups that focus more on demos, presentations, or practice you will often find the atmosphere much lighter with fewer rules.

FOR EXAMPLE:

While it is a rule to not interrupt a scene at a play party, at a demo/presentation/ practice it may be fine to ask someone who is doing something, "How do you do that?"

Rope Practice Raleigh

Fetlife Group: https://fetlife.com/groups/44047

One of the other most highly recommended groups in the area is Rope Practice. The environment is open, friendly, educational, and often free-flowing. The group meets once a month at the same location (for information join the Fetlife group for updates on events). There is a $5.00 charge per person to help support the group and cover venue costs.

The group will often have a class assigned for each meeting. These classes can range from basic knots and how to tie a rope to suspension rigging to more advanced knotwork and predicament bondage. The group welcomes presenters who have specialized skills in the art of rope or the group organizers will provide their own class instruction.

Attending the classes is highly recommended, especially if you're new, though it is not a requirement. The classes are informal and Rope Tops and Rope Bottoms will get together (either already existing partners or those willing to pair up for the classes) to learn about the topic of the meeting. It's a wonderful way to learn something new and meet new people. This is also an ideal example of the "don't interrupt a scene" rule not being applicable. A class like this openly invites questions.

Whether you're a hardcore rope fanatic/bunny or have no idea what the whole rope thing is, this is a great group. By its very nature, the group, its organizers, and its attendees are warm and welcoming and you will be sure to leave at the end of the afternoon having made some friends. Many who attend rope practice also attend other events in the area so you're 'bound' to see them again. This group also provides announcements for other activities in the area to help you navigate the local scene.

Private Meetings

These can be intimate gatherings that may cap their numbers to 20 or less or large-scale functions but, regardless of capacity, you will typically need to be a member of the group or guest of a full member in order to attend. RSVPs are usually required either by using the group/person's website, an event listing on a kink site or other means the event organizers have set forth. This is not the type of event that welcomes unregistered guests or walk-ins. The best way to get involved with such an event is to socialize with existing members (such as at munches or public events) and gain an invitation through them.

If an event-goer has invited you as their guest, whether you're their submissive or not, that person has vouched for you to the event's hosts, so be on your best behavior as it can and will reflect back on the person who invited you. It certainly doesn't take a genius to see that if someone is unhappy with your behavior at one of these private events, you will find it difficult to wrangle another invitation as no one will want to sully their own hard-earned reputation to vet you.

At these functions, you can be pretty much guaranteed to see play going on and this includes seeing people in various stages of undress. Some events are intended for all kinds of general play, and depending on the event and/or location certain play may not be allowed most often due to space or safety concern issues. If you want to play or even think you might want to do a scene, check with the group leader or location owner to find out what is considered off-limits. In fact, check with them about all of the rules ahead of time.

These private affairs tend to have fewer attendees but some can be rather large gatherings. These events are usually very informal and while you need to appear "vanilla" in your attire anywhere outside the venue, you can dress (or undress) however you feel comfortable once inside. As they are so informal and relaxed you can feel at ease to ask questions (as long as you don't interrupt a scene) or simply socialize.

Once you get involved in these types of groups your chances of finding a potential dominant further increase as you're greatly expanding your network and developing your own reputation.

Private House Party

There are some groups or sometimes "families" that periodically hold private house parties throughout the year. These are typically private events that require you to be a member or otherwise know the hosts. Since these are held at someone's private home, space can be limited and therein the attendance is often limited to a certain number. It also means you will likely receive specific instructions on parking and may even be asked to carpool to help reduce congestion on the streets and prevent potential issues with neighbors who suddenly find they have nowhere to park. In almost every instance of a private house party you must be "vanilla" attire at any point when you're outside the house, including being in the yards (unless otherwise advised), although once inside you can wear/not wear whatever you want. These are almost always play-based parties with socializing allowed in the main area. While you do not have to play to attend it is, in fact, the primary purpose of the party.

Special Events

While these are often open invitation and similar to public events, occasionally a group will organize a "special" event which can be for one day, one weekend, or even one week. In fact, the length can vary greatly depending on the event itself, although most long events will allow you the option of attending for just a couple of days if you cannot manage to schedule the full event. In almost all cases, you are required to register, RSVP, and/or purchase tickets. In some cases, when registration is required, it may mean disclosing your real name and showing identification. These large-scale events are great about discretion and you will not be addressed by your real name but it is required for age-verification and legal purposes.

Events such as these include Fetish Flea Markets now held in several states featuring weekend-long classes and shopping 'til you drop. If you're looking for a great deal on a new toy or outfit or virtually anything kinky these are the places to go. In between shopping sprees, there are a plethora of classes and demonstrations and it's a wonderful (and anonymous if you want it to be) environment to really learn. They can be expensive, especially if you have to travel and get a hotel, but they're certainly worth it for the information and product discounts you receive. These are typically held for one weekend a year, although New England Leather Alliance holds a flea market twice a year.

Other events such as Camp Crucible are a week (or more) in length and people from all walks of the lifestyle camp or lodge in cabins together. You can opt for a private arrangement or get together with a group of friends to share a spot if you don't like the idea of sleeping around a bunch of complete strangers. Everyone pitches in to help (or you can 'buy out' of doing chores), everyone is willing to impart knowledge, and everyone is willing to open up a little space for someone new. Various shows such as pony demos/parades take place and there are multiple buildings and designated dungeon spaces where play can take place virtually all day and night.

Debauchery is another weekend-long event held once a year in the southern regions. Some private facilities that usually host locally known large-scale weekend-long events can be found in many areas, but you will likely have to find your way to them by making your way through other local events before discovering who they are and how to score an invite.

Every one of these events comes with its own set of rules and expectations. They are held at all times throughout the year and you'll find that they typically are scheduled around the same time each year. That is to say, Camp Crucible will be in May every year while the New England Fetish Fair Fleamarket is in February and August, the Charlotte, NC Fleamarket is during the summer and so forth.

Find the one that best fits your time availability, finances, and abilities then go ahead and explore one. They're fine to attend as a single person or if you've begun to make contacts at this point you can try to orchestrate meeting up or carpooling together to the event. Going with others is not only fun but it can help on lowering the costs if you all agree to split expenses for room and travel.

Because these gatherings are so large you can almost always find a dedicated website where you'll find all the dates, prices, nearby hotels, FAQs, and anything else you'll need to know. This also includes what is and is not acceptable, attire rules, and general Do's and Don'ts. Many of the events will also provide you with a pre-event email or confirmation. It is highly recommended to read these as a lot of details are often provided. And read them for each event as it could change.

PUSH!

Push Your Expectations ~ Push Your Limits ~
Push Your Pleasure ~ Push Your Pain

Contact: PeteCock or SecretaryGirl via FetLife

Approximately four times a year a lovely couple puts together a large event for one evening in Durham, NC. It hosts a few DJs, bar, play space, a stage for demos and performances (ranging from singing, drag shows, and pony routines), and is a wonderful way to socialize and mingle.

The event caters to a Fetishist-type crowd and encourages leather, latex, drag, body paint, and other specialty costuming. Occasionally there will be a theme for the event where attendees are encouraged to dress in accordance with the theme although it's not required. While you needn't be decked out in leather or latex, there is a dress code and vanilla/street clothes are not allowed inside the event.

Each PUSH seems to grow and expand and always offers a unique experience. It is the type of event that people bookmark well in advance – as soon as the dates are released – and will spend lots of time (and money) finding just the perfect outfit for a night of visual and auditory stimulation that you don't find anywhere else in the local scene.

Be sure to check out their website for details, images from past events, and updates when a new date has been made available. Further, "Like" their Facebook page to make sure you get up-to-date information on events so you don't miss out.

General Meeting Rules: Regardless of whether you attend a demonstration, class, private, or public event, there are some universal rules any new submissive should be aware of to allow you continued attendance and increased reputation.

Respect the Scene/Space

The most fundamental rule in which to adhere is one I've already repeated several times but it can never be said too often and that is to never interrupt a scene. Whether you have a question about what's taking place, are uncomfortable with the scene, or are just trying to make your way from one side of the room to the other, **BE AWARE** of scenes taking place. If you have a question, wait until it's over or speak to someone in the designated social area (almost all parties have one), if you're uncomfortable then go somewhere else (i.e. social area), if you can't get to the other side then just wait.

Conversations with others should not be done near a scene. If someone strikes up a conversation with you offer to move to the side in order to continue your chat. I have mentioned this several times because this is the number one play party faux pas. Even hushed whispers can be just distracting enough to prevent someone from entering their headspace so please remember to be courteous and keep quiet. Even if you're at an event with music blasting and people talking all over the place, having a loud conversation right in the scene-space area while watching a scene can be rude and disruptive.

In addition to not interrupting a scene itself, also never interrupt aftercare. This is often an extremely emotional time for a submissive and can be a wonderfully intimate and euphoric moment. Allow the submissive **quiet** time to process and indulge in the sensations. Just because the scene ended doesn't mean you can start talking (again, take it to a social area). If you feel so inclined (i.e. the dominant is not there) you can quietly ask if they'd like some water or a blanket, but chances are the reason the dominant is not there at that moment is because they're already gathering aftercare items or clearing the scene space they just used. Wait a few moments and odds are the dominant will be there shortly. Alternatively, you can gently ask the dominant if they'd like you to clean the scene space so they can attend to their submissive more promptly. Also, whatever you do, never touch a submissive in aftercare. Generally, stay clear of any aftercare unless you've explicitly been asked for assistance.

Hands Off

Even though you're a submissive this rule still applies. Don't touch what isn't yours and/or haven't been invited to touch. This means not just toys but people too. If a dominant asks you to get such-and-such from their bag then, by all means, accommodate that dominant but do not try to be overly helpful and do so without being asked unless it's already a standing arrangement between you both. Additionally, it's good form to ask if you can hug someone and if it's another person's submissive it's appropriate to ask the dominant for permission.

Mum's the Word

Never, ever – I mean, **NEVER EVER** – talk about someone, their scene, or anything else personal outside of the event. I've already covered this in 'to out/outing' in Chapter 3 but it's such an important thing that it, too, bears repeating. If you speak to someone at an event and learn they work close to you do not ever speak to people they may know and mention you got to know them at a kinky gathering. This is 'outing' someone and it is extremely bad manners (not to mention just plain wrong) and will not do your reputation any good. DO NOT out anyone!

Cameras

DO NOT ever just snap a picture at any event whatsoever. Many events, regardless of size, length of time, or if it's privately or publicly held, will inform you right from the start or even in an email prior to the event that cameras may not be allowed at all. With camera abilities on cell phones today it makes it more difficult to prevent but if you are ever caught taking pictures or video without authorization you could find yourself in big trouble, kicked out without refund, banned from future events held by that group/person, and even shunned from the community as a whole.

If you should ever like to take a picture of someone, perhaps some wonderfully beautiful rope work, of yourself after a scene, or anything whatsoever, always ask first. Even after you've gotten the subject's permission, you do want to make an announcement to anyone near the shot or who could potentially be in the shot that you are taking a picture in order to allow them time to cover their faces or get out of the way. Also, be aware of mirrors. Many places use them and a shot near a mirror could accidentally include people who would never want their faces seen at events.

Clothing

As mentioned a few times when talking about the different types of events, most places will require that you appear "vanilla" when outside the venue or home. I also mentioned that once inside the venue/home you can be as dressed/undressed as you want, but there are a few restrictions and cleanliness rules that are often applied. First, many states and thus any venue that's considered a public space (i.e. clubs or anything other than a person's private residence) typically have a "no pink bits" rule which means that groin areas need to be covered and female nipples need to have some kind of covering – even if it's just black tape. In solidarity with the complete hypocrisy of the fact that women's nipples need to be covered but men's don't, you may see several men wearing black tape over their nipples.

Additionally, some states or cities may require g-strings, thongs, or any underwear/panties to have a certain amount of "covering" in the back. If a party states that all bottom clothing must have a 2-inch strip or greater in the back do not wear something with 1.75 inches because in some places with some authorities they are happy to find even the most insane excuse to shut events down and arrest people.

Another rule that's universal regardless of venue is don't be gross and be aware of what your body touches. If you're wearing thongs, g-strings, or nothing at all you will be required to put some type of cloth under you any time you sit. If you intend to be mostly or completely nude or bottomless, keep a small dishtowel or something similar with you at all times.

Be Helpful

Since almost all parties need to be set-up and/or broken down, it's never a bad idea to contact the organizers ahead of time and offer to help with the set-up or talk to them during the event about assisting in the break down process. They may very well decline the offer but they will remember you and appreciate it.

Along the lines of being helpful and brushing up on your general service skills, if you see an unattached dominant, if you are there by invitation of a full member, or you plan on meeting someone there who you've been speaking with, offer to get them a drink or a bite to eat. If they accept then be aware of how you "present" the items to them and put yourself in the mindset of being a submissive serving your dominant. Even if that person isn't your dominant and there's never any intention of you serving that person, it's a good opportunity to practice your service skills. Don't think about it so deeply that you overdo it but keep it in the back of your mind that this is practice for serving your dominant when the time comes.

If you're there for the express purpose of meeting a dominant, this is a prime opportunity to show your skills and attentiveness. All too often a submissive will reach the 'let's meet at this event' stage and will fail miserably. While one can understand nervousness or not having a clearly defined D/s dynamic in place at this stage, you should still be aware and provide basic service and courtesy. If their drink appears empty – offer to refresh it. If they are holding an empty plate – offer to refill it or dispose of it. If they are working an event – ask if there's anything you can do to assist. Furthermore, if the dominant does ask for assistance or does accept your offer you should follow-up throughout the event and not have your offer be a one-time deal or make them ask repeatedly for your help.

Privacy & Legalities, Scene Names, and General Information

As I've stressed throughout this book, one of the best ways to really meet the dominant you're seeking is to become active in your local community. In this lifestyle, we all understand the need for discretion as most of us need discretion for our own lives. There are far more people requiring anonymity in the lifestyle than those who are boldly proud and out loud about it, so you're in good company.

Many groups, especially munches, don't require a photo ID to attend. It is quite common and perfectly okay to use a scene name. As I touched on briefly earlier, it can be the username you have on your profile or it could be something else entirely. Many opt for a name that is vague or creatively constructed to at least "sound" vanilla versus something like "footslaveslut1234." Create a name that you will remember, respond to, and enjoy hearing. It should be a name that means something to you so you can make a connection with it and be more apt to respond when it is used. Some will opt for the easy approach and provide just their first name. No one will ask for your full name at events (beyond points mentioned below) so a first name can be a safe and easy way to introduce yourself. You could create an entirely new identity for the lifestyle (exception: see below) but that can get complicated unless you're fully committed to the new identity on a long-term basis.

The reality is that BDSM groups have to protect themselves from liability and will occasionally require photo ID, whether it's to ensure that the people attending are really who they say they are, for emergency contact information, or for age verification (that attendees are of legal age). If you're not comfortable providing that information, these meetings/events may not be the best venue for you so you may want to stick to ones like munches. However, if the munch is held at a bar or other "vanilla" facility that IDs its patrons, just be aware that you will be expected to show ID at the venue. However, you can take comfort that it's the venue looking at your ID and not the group, and the venue doesn't care why you're there, only that you're legal. If you're attending a private function held by a group/organization that may require your ID then you should have built some comfort level with those involved and trust that they will maintain your personal information in the strictest confidence.

Even within groups that require photo ID, your real name will never be used. You will be addressed by your scene name and your real identity will never be disclosed, distributed, or used for anything other than their legal protection (i.e. age verification). In most cases, you will only have to present your ID once when you first attend the group and after this confirmation then you needn't worry about flashing your license every time. Some groups may require you to redisplay your ID if they've made significant changes to their private waivers or for annual renewal purposes.

As the laws governing events, parties, and BDSM, in general, vary from state to state, some facilities may require a specific waiver. Groups that use the facilities or owners of the venue may enforce this waiver or have the right to deny you entry especially if you decline to sign the waiver. These waivers do require you to initial and/or sign your legal name and it will often be checked against your photo ID for verification. Once more, the facilities or groups utilizing the facility will often keep these papers locked away and they are not for release, public display, or in any way shared unless a legal request has been made (possibly by subpoena).

Meeting in public provides everyone a safe environment, with no need to worry about anyone accidentally overhearing kinky-talk, as everyone is there for the same reason (and most groups are given a private room for such things as munches), and you get to have that face-to-face interaction that's so much more satisfying than random emails. If you don't find the one dominant you really want to submit to, you might meet someone who can introduce you to them down the road. If nothing else, you will often wind up making some really great friends.

Approach these get-togethers with the idea of making friends and networking, of learning more about the lifestyle, styles of playing/scening, and general D/s interactions. Do not go into them thinking you're going to hook-up because that's not the purpose of these meetings. Thinking like this will probably disappoint and frustrate you and you'll likely drop out of the group. Plus, as "they" say, the best things come when you are not trying so hard to find them. The less you focus on finding a dominant the greater the chance that you'll wind up meeting them... when you least expect it.

Regardless of what venue you pick to attend, you should be friendly and outgoing instead of being a wallflower. Going anywhere for the first time, surrounded by strangers, can be very daunting, but just keep telling yourself these people are there to socialize and you are all there for the same reasons. Even if you can't go up to people and initiate a conversation, smile and keep your body language open and relaxed. If someone notices that you seem shy but look like you want to be a part of things, they will come up to you. You can also contact the group leaders before the gathering and let them know that you are looking forward to attending but you don't know anyone. Often they will be happy to greet you and make some introductions to help break the ice.

Chapter 18

Personal Grooming

I'm placing this chapter here before discussing meeting a dominant in person for a "date" (although these tips should be standard before attending any social event) because, while how you present yourself online is important, how you present yourself in real life is even more important. Not only are you trying to win people over with your charm and personality, but physical appearance can also be equally important, especially during the first meeting.

Personal grooming can be thought of in two ways:

1. Your own personal grooming and hygiene
2. Learning how to personally groom your dominant (sometimes called body service)

I'm sorry to disappoint you but this chapter is dedicated to the former and while you might think this shouldn't need to be covered, it has been proven on far too many occasions that it really does. Whether you think you have personal grooming down or not, you should, at the very least, give this chapter a quick once-over as you may actually discover you might not be as adept as you originally thought. After all, enough instances have arisen both on and offline to prompt this chapter in the first place.

While we typically feel that women have personal grooming down to a science, they are not exempt from some of the issues mentioned in this chapter.

There are a surprising number of submissives who either don't care or don't realize that their appearance can be just as, or in some cases, even more off-putting than any lascivious email. Whatever the excuse for previous poor grooming, this section is meant to help you take a closer look at yourself (something you should get used to doing as a submissive anyway) and realize what areas could use a complete change or, at the very least, a little tweak. While you needn't be the next Don Juan/Supermodel or maintain an expensive wardrobe, some small attention to personal details can go a long way.

Why Is Your Personal Appearance Important?

First, it makes you more physically appealing. While many will say physicality doesn't matter, there is some level of physical attraction that plays a role for most people but that doesn't mean everyone finds the same things attractive. Some may swoon over a well-muscled man or woman, others may find muscles on any gender to be the opposite of sexy. Some love robust and curvy figures while others love lithe forms. Whatever it might be, there is some aspect of physical attraction that often draws us to someone enough to want to engage in communication. No matter how much someone may love your mind, sense of humor, or anything else about you, there often needs to be some type of physical attraction to spark desire. So much of this lifestyle is based on sensuality and allure and not finding someone physically appealing takes some of the fun and heat out of play, so yes, being physically attractive is important even if it's not the most important aspect. While this is a seemingly 'superficial' attitude, the fact is that it is human nature to opt for the physically or sexually appealing first. There are many who love all body types or will casually play with a great many people without caring about physicality because they are there to do a scene and that's the only 'connection' they need, but when we're talking about finding someone with whom you want to be serious and establish something long-term, attraction comes into play. If you're smelly, disheveled, or even creepy looking many dominants won't go near you, especially when play/scenes are intended to be intimate.

Second, when you are in service to someone, you are a reflection of them. A submissive appearing somewhere disheveled may be cute or funny in a "just been used" way, but a chronic habit of it means that you don't care about yourself. If you don't care about yourself how can you care for your dominant or care about how others may perceive the dominant through you? Whether you notice or not, if others don't want to be around you, it could affect your dominant's reputation and general acceptance amongst lifestyle peers. Now, for that to happen we're talking about some extremely poor hygiene and appearance, but unfortunately, the lifestyle isn't immune to those who seem to have these issues.

Tanning: Even those who appear extremely well-groomed need to be wary. If you are fastidious about your appearance that's wonderful, but take a moment to ask yourself, "Do I think something looks sexy but could really be silly?"

A great example of this is tanning (self or natural). Just as many men do this as women and the results vary greatly. If you have it down to an art and get that beautiful light glow in the off-season and a deep luscious tan during the summer, good for you, skip ahead. However, if you have that dark tan all year then chances are you look a little silly or somewhat out of place unless you live somewhere that's generally warm/sunny all year. If your tan is really just orange paint on your skin, you're guaranteed to look like an Oompa Loompa, and that's not a compliment. Watch out for artificial tanning options like spray-tan or lotions as they can become uneven, orange, or even leave nasty weird coloring on your hands.

If you insist on tanning, then go with seasonal-appropriate tones and adjust accordingly. Talk with someone at a spa or tanning facility about what's appropriate for the time of year and your own physical make-up. A naturally ghost-white redhead may look bad with anything beyond just a little coloring whereas someone who has dark hair or olive complexion could do well with dark tones to really accent their other features.

Clothes: It's okay to find an actor or even a character who has a style that you really like and to emulate it whenever possible. Back in the 90s "The Rachel" hairstyle was all the rage while not long ago the "Guido" look was alarmingly popular because of *Jersey Shore*. So much of our wardrobe and accessories come from celebrities which is why they're used so often for marketing and branding purposes. It's absolutely fine to follow a trend or to mimic a style, just remember not to get lost in it to the point where you're trying to be exactly like the person/character and have no sense of self or personal style anymore.

The most important thing is to dress to suit your body type, in clothes that make you feel comfortable and that fit properly. While it's perfectly acceptable to follow a trend, don't feel like you have to rely on them and remember it's more important to be yourself and be comfortable. It's also okay to have a couple of different looks such as "business" style, "casual," "kinky," and even outright "sexy."

I know most men hate to shop and once they know their sizes they just go to the store, pick up something that looks appealing, match the size, and check out. I am guilty of this myself on several occasions. Regardless of gender though, there's the reality that if you want to find clothes that match your body type and fit properly, you will actually have to bite the bullet and try on some things in the store. Different labels and styles have size variations so just because you're size X normally, those jeans you just picked up may not fit as well as they should because the brand uses a different "interpretation" of sizes. For those who typically don't like to shop, now's the time to get used to shopping since dominants may enjoy it and want you to accompany them on excursions or, alternatively, the dominant may hate it and leave it to you to run to the store. Get used to looking carefully at what's on the racks and shelves, gauge prices and bargains, and learn to use the fitting rooms.

Remember, try to have a pair of shoes that can work with each of your outfits. Wearing a pair of sneakers with a suit is generally not recommended, although in certain (very select) circumstances this could be pulled off and look good. Further, try to keep at least one pair of sneakers designated for when you go out versus every-day-use so they don't look ragged. A pair of boots and a pair of dress shoes with a generic color (to match with most outfits) can complement most outfits.

Hair: Hair can be a very personal issue. People will notice your hair and how it's maintained and styled. If you're a bald guy, you're pretty much worry-free, but if you're nearly bald, avoid a comb-over at all costs. Keep it neatly trimmed or consider buzzing/shaving what's left. Bald is and can be very sexy so if you're facing hair loss put some thought into this option.

If you have long hair make sure it's well-maintained. Natty, ratty, tangled, and straw-like long hair is visually unappealing and certainly won't invoke the image of a dominant's hands wrapped in those luscious locks. Whether you keep it loose, pulled back, or otherwise styled, make sure your face isn't covered and it should be trimmed to keep it fresh looking.

This could mean investing in some hair care products to help manage those tresses but it doesn't mean you have to break the bank or fill an entire bathroom with products. If you're a guy with long hair but you're not really sure about what products to use to help maintain it you should speak with a stylist, a hairdresser, friend, or even look online, for some recommendations about conditioning and maintenance.

Short hair should be kept neat and that awkward period when your hair is just long enough for a haircut should let you know it's time to schedule an appointment. If your budget allows for it, it's a good idea to set up regularly scheduled appointments with a barber or hairdresser, and many places will ask you as you're checking out if you'd like to schedule your next appointment. If possible, take advantage of this and maintain a reasonable hair care regiment.

A note about hair length: Whatever your hair length or style is right now, keep it that way but do realize that some dominants may enjoy controlling how their submissive keeps their hair. Some may like guys with close-cropped styles, some love the fades, others love guys with long hair. Some love women with a bob, while others may want you to grow out your hair as long as possible, while others may want you to just maintain something just below the shoulders. Just be aware that there are plenty of dominants who enjoy this level of control and will tell you what length, color, and style they prefer and may even go so far as to require specific hair care regiments.

Hair Product: Whatever the length or style of your hair, avoid using so much product that your dominant's hand could get stuck in it or can't even break through the shell if they go to stroke or take you by the hair. You should also try to avoid using so many types of product that your bathroom looks like it exploded with products. This is especially true if you ever become a live-in servant as the space allotted for your belongings might be limited.

If you find you need to use an excessive amount of product to create your 'look,' it might be time to try other brands or perhaps explore alternative styles. A single more expensive product may hold better and take the place of needing multiple cheaper products. Remember, you can always speak to your barber or hairdresser for suggestions, but take note that they often have specific products they are going to try to sell regardless of what's really best for your style and budget. Most of those products can be found cheaper through other brands or even at different locations like hair and make-up discount retailers.

If you go to a cheap chain place, you likely won't find the advice you need so it might be worth a one-time splurge to try a more high-end salon to get a good style, some advice, and possibly some products.

Facial Hair: While this is typically geared towards men, there are women who have some facial hair. This is also a matter of personal taste whether you have any or none at all. Once again, I say whatever you're doing with it now, keep doing it and once things get more serious with your potential dominant you can discuss if they want you to do something different once you submit to them. This could be wanting a man to be smooth shaven or wanting the woman to leave whatever hair she has alone and let it go natural or vice versa.

If you're shaving use a moisturizer (discussed in further detail below) and this goes for any gender as shaving can cause rough skin – this is especially true in winter/colder seasons and if you don't normally shave your face. If you do maintain facial hair make sure that it is neat looking either by keeping it trimmed or at least combed. If you do have a beard, stay away from something that makes you look crazed, like a hobo, or generally unkempt. Many stores, even grocery stores, will sell trimmers, scissors, combs, and other supplies to help you maintain whatever facial hair you have in whatever style you want.

Remember, if you have any type of facial hair and you're eating or drinking, be more diligent about wiping your face as the hair is prone to catching crumbs and droplets. In fact, regardless of facial hair, you should get into the habit of gently wiping your mouth after every (or every other) bite and that means using a napkin, not your hands or sleeves.

One area of facial hair that's frequently overlooked is the eyebrows. Do note that eyebrows are plural… yes, you are supposed to have two of them. The unibrow is not attractive and should be avoided at all costs. Ensuring there is a space between them doesn't mean just trimming the hair in the middle, but keeping it hairless.

Wildly bushy eyebrows also detract from your appearance and should be trimmed and kept even. Most hair/nail salons or even mall kiosks offer eyebrow waxing, plucking, or threading services or get some small scissors, razor, or tweezers and do it yourself. This means taming even just one or two wayward strands. Alternatively, having your eyebrows worked until they're just a thin line could be equally unattractive.

Also, regardless of gender, you should pick up a nose hair trimmer. Seeing a bush in someone's nose is so unappealing I can assure you most dominants will desire that this area is properly maintained. Some will use cuticle scissors and while this is fine there is a chance at nicking yourself and not getting a nice even clip. They're relatively inexpensive to begin with but don't go too cheap or they won't actually cut the hairs. Remember, just maintain the rim of your nostrils and keep it from having hairs sticking out; you shouldn't be sticking it up your nose. Not only is it not safe or hygienic but those hairs are also there to help protect you from particles including those that can make you sick.

Check your ears for hair and wax. Some folks, particularly men, have hairy ears so make sure you maintain this area as well whether you do it at home or have it done with your regular haircut. Seeing a chunk of ear wax pushing its way out of someone's ear is just gross and it's such a simple thing to do to keep them clean. If, for whatever reason, you are not in the habit of cleaning them out after each shower now's the time to get into that habit.

Body/Genital Hair: Once again, whatever your current habits are you should continue with them until you connect with a dominant, but this is an area that many dominants like to have a say in, especially the hair around the genitals. Regardless of what a potential dominant may desire, whether it's maintaining a little body/genital hair, being wild and bushy, or completely smooth, it's a good idea to still maintain a groomed appearance.

If you are truly a grizzly man with hair that pours out over your shirt, some trimming may be in order, if only to stop it from sprouting out of your clothes. This may require enlisting the help of a friend to get your back and any other hard-to-reach places. While you don't have to cut it down to stubble you should at least be able to wear clothes without looking like you're also wearing a fur coat. Also, if you're extra hairy you may also be prone to extra sweating. Be aware of this and adjust the use of deodorant accordingly.

Some love bushy genital areas on men and women, some love women to have a little strip or even a design for their pubic hair, while others love the absolutely smooth front and back for any gender. Being completely smooth may require shaving (perhaps daily) or getting waxed. If you are a pretty hairy person and are tired of shaving your entire body every day, then waxing may be the best method as it lasts significantly longer. For those so inclined and with the financial resources, exploring laser hair removal treatment might be an option. You can look at spot treatments such as just that fuzz above your lip or see if there's a reduced fee for doing nearly your whole body. Be aware that some dominants might even want (regardless of gender) legs, armpits, and even forearms to be hairless as well.

Now's the time to get over any personal shyness regarding your body, especially genitals. If you cannot maintain a regiment yourself due to the frequency it may require or an inability to reach certain areas, it could mean putting yourself on display for a friend or professional through salons.

Cologne/Perfumes/Scented Products: We've all had someone walk by, have been in an elevator, or in some way encountered someone who either had excessive body odor that made you want to gag or had excessive cologne/perfume that made you want to gag.

Cologne/Perfume is a very personal choice and what might smell utterly delicious on one person can be either virtually non-existent or foul on someone else. This is due to body chemistry and, as you know, everyone's is different, so take the time to explore different scents. Don't just use the spray testing card at the store but give yourself a little spritz to see how it truly smells once it mixes with your body. This doesn't mean you should spray every kind of cologne on every open space of your body in one day. It means to take a few days and try a few that seem to really appeal to you. Ask the clerk which ones seem to be the most popular, especially ones that seem to be popular with the purchaser's partners. Ask friends to give you some honest feedback. A good indicator will be when people just naturally say, "Oh, wow you smell so good."

You should have a few colognes/perfumes to match the seasons and daily activity. Most people can't afford to use that $100 bottle of cologne/perfume on just going to the gym, so a body spray that's reasonably priced may be ideal for the everyday grind and then reserve those most expensive bottles for events and special occasions. In fact, some of the scents that can typically be pricey may have cheaper alternatives. While not expensive, an example would be the Ed Hardy line – which usually sells for around $20-$30 (although they used to be more expensive) but they also have a cheaper body spray that's only about $8-$10.

I wear Dolce & Gabbana Light Blue and Ed Hardy for spring and summer and Aspen, Diesel, and John Varvatos for the fall and winter. For everyday 'putzing' around, I use a body spray since its cheap and it smells good, and that way I won't have to blast through my more expensive colognes. For extra special occasions (i.e. weddings) I wear Mont Blanc regardless of the season. I'll wear Tim McGraw's cologne or True Religion for most events. I continually get reactions that range from, "Oh, you smell so good," to, on one occasion, outright mauling (in a fun way).

There are plenty of options for perfumes and colognes and even more options for body sprays – although these seem to be mostly available to women. Don't forget, however, there's also scented lotions and scented hair care products. People are often drawn to attractive scents, however, do be aware that some people are highly sensitive and scents can cause allergic reactions. For the most part, use your lotions, perfumes, colognes, and such sparingly, and it's okay to get one of the travel-sized options to bring with you to places in case you need a quick refresher.

The Key: Never have people know you've arrived before you even get through the door.

Deodorant: In direct relation to scents and smelling good... Deodorant... USE IT! Unless you and the dominant you're hoping to meet have a fetish for natural body musk, you should be using deodorant. Whether you select scented or unscented, you will want to focus on which gives you the best protection. If you opt for a scented brand make sure it matches or complements the other scents you use so you don't become a headache-inducing cluster of clashing scents. Many perfumes/colognes come in box sets that allow you to have the body wash, cologne, and deodorant to make sure your scent matches, so while they may seem a little costly you are getting a good set and investing in one of these might be a good idea. Some stores offer great deals on sets whether it's getting additional items or even a complimentary gift, but don't feel like you have to get the box set for each and every one of your scents. Just one box set of one of your favorite or most frequently used scent should be all you need and it will help prevent a clash of scents from overwhelming those around you.

Alternatively, there are always those few who reach up to give you a hug and you're almost knocked over by the stench coming from them. Events can tend to generate excessive heat from the number of people in an enclosed space and that causes many to sweat more than normal. Most people will respond by opting for a handshake or a drive-by pat on the back on their way by if you've been labeled as one of *those* stinky people. Even if you and/or your dominant have a scent/natural musk fetish you may need to concede to some protection for the benefit of others and the ability to be close to people while socializing.

Lip/Skin Care: Regardless of gender, you should be aware that certain parts of the body tend to get dry or rough and may need some attention. Typically the elbows are the most common areas on everyone's body that get ashy or rough, especially in the colder months. Lotions and moisturizers come in a huge variety of options and sizes so you can keep a large one at home and a travel-sized one in your car or at work. Sometimes you might have to apply lotion every single day, other times you may need it every few days. Whatever your body needs, get in the habit of giving this oft-overlooked area a little attention.

Feet can get incredibly dry, cracked, and calloused and definitely could use attention. Regardless of gender, if your feet are on the rough end it might be worth a trip to the local nail salon and ask for a pedicure. They will usually soak your feet, clip your nails, file off the rough skin, apply some lotion, and even give a little massage. If you want to have your nails painted it's typically included or you can opt out of this portion. Otherwise, it's a good idea to maintain a moisturizing regiment for your feet and this can be great practice for you serving your dominant. Some people are adamantly opposed to feet so if touching someone else's feet in service such as this, then be sure to mention that in your profile or early on in conversation because many dominants love to have their feet rubbed whether it's just to relax or if you are to moisturize their feet as well. Many dominants and submissives have a foot fetish which could include pampering such as this to full on licking and sucking, to wanting to have them rest their feet on your body. If this is something that interests both of you then providing this service can be fun and exciting.

If it's a huge gross-out factor for you then you might want to consider a dominant who doesn't care about having this type of service done. Regardless, you should still be in the habit of taking care of your own feet so they don't look like troll feet or feel like sandpaper

Another popular part of the body that often gets overlooked but can also get rough are the lips. If you plan on kissing your dominant, whether on their lips, hands, feet, or any other body parts, don't do it with rough, cracked, split, or harsh lips. A little lip balm goes a long way and it doesn't matter whether you get it from your nearby dollar store, grocery store, or expensive spa-like shop. The thing that does matter is that you remember to use it. There are also lip glosses which add a little color or sheen to the lips while also giving them a little moisture – and some even have different flavors. Keeping a lip gloss or just plain chapstick on hand is always a good idea. If you have a chronic condition or are exposed to the elements, you may find the traditional sticks ineffective. Have no fear! Neosporin lip treatment is supposed to work wonders. No matter how smooth or chapped your lips are, pay attention to them.

Whether you are using lotion on a specific area like your hands, elbows, face, or feet or you use it for your whole body, there are scented and unscented options. Some are scented to assist with relaxation, some are scented to just smell nice, while unscented is a good option across the board. In fact, even if you don't think you really need it, it's not a bad idea to lotion-up your hands periodically so that they're soft or gentle to the touch when you caress your dominant or when your dominant wants to caress you.

General Hygiene

WASH… YOUR… HANDS!

Yes, this apparently still needs to be addressed. You should be washing your hands every time you use the bathroom. Everything you touch in a restroom, whether in a public place or the one at home, is filthy and we absolutely don't want your disgusting hands on us, touching our glasses/plates, or handling any food we will eat without washing your hands. Be aware of the restroom door. If it pushes open, then use your elbow or foot to push the door open. If it has a handle that requires you to pull it open, grab an extra paper towel and use that to hold the handle.

Everyone before you who didn't wash their hands will have touched the door handle and so touching it on your way out will just completely negate any hand-washing you just did.

Even though you should already be washing your hands with some frequency you should still pay attention to your nails. While it's understandable to have dirty nails after a hard day's work regardless of what kind of business you're in, it's unattractive to see grit and grime embedded in and around your nails when you're going out. This isn't an issue restricted to just men because I have encountered many women who have worked all day with grit under their nails or that you're unable to tell if they're dirty because they're polished over. If you work in a field that's especially dirty or prone to potential hazards like construction, animal care, or medical fields then you should invest in a specialized hand cleanser. Get a manicure kit – there are those sold toward women and toward men but it shouldn't matter as they mostly have the same core items. Get into the habit of scraping under your nails. DO NOT BITE YOUR NAILS or cuticles. Keep in mind that some dominants may want you to maintain your nails at a certain length such as women having long nails as a dominant might just enjoy the visual of them or might enjoy feeling them gently stroking their skin or even feeling them sink into them during the height of passion. Both women and men might be told to keep their nails cut and trimmed as the dominant might want you to please them with your fingers inside their anus or vagina and they don't want to get nicked.

Most people do not find farting or hocking a loogie in any way amusing or attractive. If you need to blow your nose, spit up, clear phlegm, or relieve yourself in any way then ask to be excused and use the restroom or another room. This also means do not pick your nose or constantly sniff back mucus. The latter is something many people do without even noticing it and it can be incredibly annoying to those around you so try to be aware of your actions and just use a tissue.

Men - keep your hands off your crotch. We know it's there, you know it's there, it's not going anywhere, so just stop. If you're truly that unadjusted in your drawers or you're a trans man who wears a packer or similar equipment that might be slipping then, once more, excuse yourself to the bathroom and adjust. If we see you constantly scratching at it we will assume you have something unpleasant going on and most dominants will give you a wide berth.

With all that said, it really boils down to my favorite thing - some common sense — along with some common courtesy and just plain common decency. Many times it's an unconscious thought/habit or maybe an area of grooming you never really considered in the past. Now it's written out for you, plain and clear, so start paying attention to yourself in acute detail because you can be sure we are paying attention, and the more of a mess you look and act the less likely you will be able to find a willing dominant.

Chapter 19

Non-Verbal Communication

I want to discuss two aspects of Non-Verbal Communication in this chapter. While I have separated them into *Body Language* and *Social Cues*, they are often interchangeable or in conjunction with one another.

Learn to Read... Body Language

We all do things subconsciously with our body that can tell a story. It is not an art but, rather, a science to learn how to read what the body is really saying, and this knowledge has been used by profilers and law enforcement officers for years to discern when suspects might be lying. More recently, technology has been developed to gauge physiological responses when someone is asked questions or put into certain scenarios. While we don't have to take it that far, it is important for you, the submissive, to recognize, read, interpret, and respond to your dominant's body language. It is also important that you're aware of what your own body language can be saying to observers and to perhaps even adjust your behavior.

First and foremost, you will need to take situations and context into consideration. Remember that you will be primarily interacting with people who are at events, parties, or have been/will be playing. You may also be too new to know anything about the other guests or their habits. While it is important to be aware of body language – what your own body is projecting to others as well as reading what others may be projecting – don't become so consumed with trying to read intent that you inadvertently come across as a stalker. Don't announce that you're reading body language. This will make people very uncomfortable and they will become self-conscious. Not only is it uncool to make others uncomfortable but now everyone will be on guard and you'll never get a genuine reading from them again. You'll likely find yourself pushed out of chat-circles and discussions or just ignored.

Personal Space: Invasion of personal space depends entirely on context. Someone who enters another's personal space can be expressing interest, seeking intimacy, or engaging in quiet/intimate conversation. In most instances, this is a welcome breech of your/their personal space, especially if you have established some level of trust. Alternatively, there's the "creepy invader." This is someone who has complete disregard for, or is absolutely clueless about, the boundaries of personal space. This is a person who will inch into the "circle" you've created to be included in your conversation or be needlessly close to you. You can get a "vibe" as to the intent of the invasion and go with your gut instinct.

Head Position: A cocked head could indicate that someone is interested in what you're saying. In some cases, a bowed or lowered head could indicate secretiveness. However, given that we're dealing with kink we will have to consider if the person is a submissive and, therein, a lowered gaze or head could indicate respect, humility, or be a directive from their dominant. If a dominant's head is lowered while chatting with others this may be more of an indicator of disinterest or furtiveness.

Eyes: This works in conjunction with head position. Someone who is engaged in your conversation will lock eyes with either your eyes or your mouth. Some people will watch the mouth more often as a means to help "hear" better, especially when at a loud or crowded event. Avoiding eye contact entirely can be an indication of avoidance or disinterest but, again, if they are a submissive this could also be a restriction put on them by a dominant or a sign of respect.

The look in a person's eyes can also be a clear indicator. A dilated pupil could indicate interest in what you're saying or even attraction. It could also mean the person is under the influence and while this may not be the case since alcohol/drugs are not allowed at most parties or events the person may have 'indulged' before they entered. Still, you can (or should be able to) usually tell when someone has "checked-out" by a distant, foggy, or vacant look in their eyes.

The direction a person's eyes shift when asked a question will indicate if they're thinking or lying. Right-handed people will often move their eyes to the left if they're trying to recall something and move their eyes to the right if they're lying. Conversely, left-handed people's eyes will usually move to the right if they're attempting to remember and to the left if they're lying. Another good eye indicator of lies is a more rapid pace of blinking.

Another eye cue is the partially lowered lid, a mini-squint. It could indicate the person doesn't agree with something you said but may not be willing to confront you or what you've said has bothered them in some way. Alternatively, it could mean they're trying to hear you better or decipher something you said or it could even indicate they're skeptical about something you said. Figuring out the specific intention might mean using those other context clues but if you see someone squinting it should be some cue for you that one of these things is happening and you will need to assess the intent.

Shifting eyes can be a "tell" on what's going on with a person. Looking at their phone, the clock, or their watch with some frequency might mean they need to get somewhere or want to walk away but don't want to interrupt you if you're in the middle of speaking. If their eyes drift around the room or keep going back to a spot or to someone in particular, it could mean they are done with the conversation or bored or someone else is trying to get their attention and they're trying not to be rude by interrupting you. This could be a sign that you are monopolizing the person's time, have talked their ear off, or have just outright bored them but they're too polite to say anything. If their attention is wandering in any capacity, take this as being the same thing as them verbally saying: "I'm done with this conversation."

Smile: People have many smiles in their repertoire. As just a few examples there's the "Cheese" smile that gets plastered on when a picture is taken, the half-smile that could indicate they're placating you but don't really find you funny, and the genuine smile. It may be difficult to discern the differences in a person you've just met so it might require several meetings before you can begin to determine how many smiles the person has and their meanings, but other times you can get a general "feel" for the intention if you are paying attention.

Stance: A person with a relaxed stance is someone who is open to communication, not lying, and is, in general, having a good time. A person who fidgets could be lying, hiding something, or might just be anxious. Fidgeting can also be the result of aches and pains so know a little about someone before declaring the person a big liar. Again, context clues are a big help here because someone who is fidgeting or seems nervous could be brand new to the scene and might be overwhelmed or shy. Someone who turns their body away from you, especially if you're trying to speak to them one-on-one, could easily be indicating they're disinterested or might not even like you but doesn't want a confrontation. Someone with folded arms can be closed off to communication, doesn't want to be bothered, and is sending out a 'do not approach' signal. Crossed arms could also just be a comfortable stance so read other signals that could assist you in determining if this is a stance of comfort or a 'back off' alert.

When sitting, you can determine if someone is leaning back and appears comfortable and open or if they're leaning forward toward you. Either can be a good sign that the person is interested or willing to engage in chit-chat. A relaxed appearance can show they're open, comfortable and relaxed while speaking to you, while a forward lean could mean they're very interested in what you're saying. However, you will want to watch for a rigid sitting position. While some dominants expect or enforce good posture from their submissives one can usually determine if this is the case, if the person might just have back pain and is trying to relieve the tension, or is genuinely not interested in you. Watch for the turned-away position even while someone is sitting.

Voice: At events, some people are just excited, some are in sub-space, and others are in aftercare or coming out of it. Any of these could alter the manner in which a person speaks. Some people speak with a naturally slow and controlled voice while others are more hyper or naturally animated. Once you can determine what their "normal" patterns are you can begin to discern what abnormal voice changes can indicate. Someone who normally speaks in an average voice or pace may suddenly speed up if they're excited or agitated. They may slow down if they're angry, lost in thought, lying, or trying to emphasize a point.

Listen for excessive detail or lots of exaggeration as well. You may encounter someone trying to sound better, bigger, more skillful, more popular, or someone who is over-inflating a story to sound cool. People exaggerate all the time. "Oh man that thing weighed a ton. I couldn't believe I had to carry it." Another good example of common exaggeration would be: "I had to take like a gazillion calls." The word choice indicates a playful and obvious overstatement. "It sounded like a herd of elephants," or "It felt like being hit with a baseball bat." We know there were no elephant herds and that they weren't hit with a bat, it's storytelling language meant to enhance the experience.

Untruthful exaggeration is often easy to spot and, essentially, is a lie. Some people feel that inflating events makes them sound more believable or more amazing but it discredits them and puts them in a poor light. This is the person who says, "I fought 30 guys at the bar. No really, dude, seriously, there was like 30 of them." He is insistent on this number as being an actual fact and let's be realistic, even Chuck Norris would have a hard time with 30 guys in a bar fight.

This could be someone who needs to impress an audience with their knowledge, making it appear they are better versed in a subject than they are in reality. Another good indicator of the exaggerated liar is someone who changes the details depending on who they tell or when they tell the story. It's entirely possible that you've heard a tale from someone with one set of details but 3 months later the person doesn't remember they told you and now you're hearing it with a completely different set of details. While memory gets a little skewed over time and there might be slight or inconsequential variations, odds are, if the significant details vary from each telling it's likely a made-up story from a poor liar.

They say: "The truth of the lie is in the details." Someone who is trying to convince you of something, but is lying, will often use an overabundance of detail. Don't confuse this with a good storyteller. "Painting a scene" in words requires a good deal of detail. It's often easy to tell the two apart.

Evasive Language: If you say: "I heard you were involved with…" (any person, subject, or job for example) and the response is: "Who told you that?" this could mean one of two things. If you say it to a relative stranger it could come off as you being creepy and the person will genuinely want to know who is sharing personal information. It could also be deflective or evasive language. Nothing is admitted or denied and they have altered the course of the conversation away from specifics about them to focus on where you got the information.

If you were to ask: "What happened when x, y, z happened?" And they respond: "Well, depends on what you *mean* by x, y, x," or "What do *you* think happened?" They are, once more, deflecting the conversation. It's entirely possible that the person doesn't feel comfortable speaking to you about the subject, that they don't want to have this conversation in such a public setting, or they don't know you that well and there is no established rapport. Again, context clues are important, but if you feel the question you asked is fairly basic or if it's someone you're meeting up with and the point is to speak to each other in person and they're being evasive by giving non-answers or redirecting this could be a warning bell.

Everything is subjective. Don't rely entirely on body language but do be aware of it. This will help you determine if you have caught someone's attention or have lost it completely. It will help you decide if someone does or does not like you regardless of reason. It will also help you become a better listener and to make your own body language more open and thus be more approachable. Given the environment that you are entering (the lifestyle) there are some protocols you will have to allow for, such as those I've mentioned where dominants might have standing orders with their submissives or some dominants (albeit extremely rare) might simply not want to engage in conversation with any submissives.

Also remember, since most of your interactions will be at social events and parties, people behave differently depending on whether they're in large groups, small groups, with close friends, or one-on-one. People will reveal different levels of themselves within these various circles and, given the nature of the lifestyle, some will always remain cordial but distant at events as they simply don't want to get too close to folks who could potentially out them. While they're comfortable with friendship being at events-only, their body language will indicate their disinterest in opening up further.

Keep your questions and conversation light and casual. Speaking in a crass or demeaning way to anyone, and especially a dominant, could be very off-putting and might even get you uninvited from future events. Asking people what they do for a living or where they live could cause them to lock down. Let relationships build naturally.

Social Cues – Don't Be "That" Guy/Girl

Social cues are very similar to body language and some ability to read that language will help you to pick up on specific social cues. Ignoring these cues often leads to social faux pas. While everyone makes mistakes, especially when navigating a new community, you can avoid some of these pitfalls.

It is important to remember that even though you're at an event and one of the main purposes is to mix and mingle, there are still cliques. While this isn't a high school flashback with the "cool kids" making fun of or excluding everyone else, it is, however, a natural social occurrence. It develops as people begin to get closer – everyone has those with whom they feel super close and will socialize outside of lifestyle events, friends who they will do things with only occasionally, social or event-only friends, and some they just don't like. While many folks are inclusive and open to people coming and going during conversations because they realize they are, in fact, in a public space, there are the occasional instances when a couple or group of people engage in private conversations. Being attuned to social cues and body language will help you avoid walking into those awkward moments and, also help you get out of them just as easily.

With some insight into body language and social cues you can determine by the way people are positioned and how they appear to be speaking if the conversation is private. People huddled closely together, speaking in hushed tones, or with intense or serious looks on their faces are typically having a private conversation. You may find an exception to this if you find those huddled close together and talking quietly because they're being respectful of a scene and aren't, necessarily, engaged in a private conversation upon which you shouldn't infringe.

FOR EXAMPLE:

At an event, three or four people were standing together but off to the side having a private conversation. A younger man who has been to numerous events in the past but has proved to be blind to social cues and body language erred once more. He walked into the group and all conversation stopped and all eyes turned toward him. Most people would understand that they've walked into something, apologize, and walk away. He commented, "Oh, seems like I walked into a private conversation, it's okay, go ahead," and then continued to stand there.

This young man was not really friends with anyone, always drifting on the outskirts of friendships and was, to many, someone people were friendly with strictly at events. Having no established relationships with anyone involved, it was beyond presumptuous for him to expect a private conversation to continue in his presence. What's more, he even acknowledged he walked into a private conversation. The right thing to do would be to either keep on walking and not interrupt the group or quickly apologize and leave.

When engaged in a conversation, people will indicate if they're willing to keep talking or if you will only be privy to small talk. They will speak in general terms if they want to finish or convey a thought or statement but don't intend to elaborate. Essentially, they may give you a courtesy response but have no intention of getting into anything personal. Pushing for more information can create an awkward moment. Remember that you will not be granted an 'all-access pass' to people's lives just because you're at the same event or even had a scene with them. This lifestyle calls for a great deal of discretion, so while people may speak generally about themselves few will divulge actual details until a firmly established relationship/friendship has been developed.

FOR EXAMPLE:

If you ask a dominant, "So, what do you do for work?" and they answer something generalized or vague like, "I'm in IT," this isn't an invitation to push by asking, "Oh, for what company?" If they wanted to share that information they would have responded, "I do IT support for such-and-such company."

While the dominant might seem uninterested in providing details that doesn't mean it has to be the end of your conversation. Especially if this is a dominant you're interested in or have made plans to meet up with at an event to see how well you click in real life. If they've given you a vague-like answer you could simply say: "Oh, I've always found that field interesting, but it's beyond my understanding," laugh it off and move on to the next subject. This should be an indication to you that personal questions may not be appropriate at this time so, instead, try to swing the conversation into more neutral territory. If you aren't shy, feel free to provide some information about yourself. If a person feels that you are open about yourself they may slowly start to share more about themselves in return.

Remember that some people have known each other for a long time and have established relationships outside of events. Many lifestyle friendships become real-life ones with shared outside interests. We hang out, go to dinner, watch movies, and do any number of other things together. Inside jokes and camaraderie are built over time and lead to the relationships you see. Do not expect to be privy to these types of relationships immediately, so just go slow and steady and develop personal bonds on your own and in their own time. Sometimes you will get lucky by becoming friends with someone who has a good group of established friends or who is otherwise well-known within the community and you will gain friendships more rapidly through them, but don't expect this to the norm, don't expressly single out someone you feel is popular for the purposes of using their popularity for your own gain, and don't assume that just because a person you've become friends with is popular others will open up to you immediately.

FOR EXAMPLE:

Seeing people tickle or fondle each other does not mean you have an open invitation to do the same. There was at least one person who didn't understand this in a local community and would often see 'horsing around' amongst friends and assume that because he 'knew' them too he was allowed to engage in such horsing around.

Some people will use terms that might be pet names or special names that are only used by close friends. Do not think that because someone is called one thing by their friends that you have the liberty to do the same. This type of scenario can be difficult to decipher since the lifestyle itself is based on people using titles and pseudonyms. Paying attention to social cues and body language can help you determine if this is how the person should be addressed in general or if it is a playful term developed within a close relationship. If you're unsure how the person wishes to be addressed you should simply ask, "I heard so-and-so call you such-and-such. Is that how you like to be addressed?" In most cases, the person will be happy to inform you if that is correct or if it was something reserved for friends-only.

Those who are genuine friends have been made privy to private information. They may know each other's real names, where they work, phone numbers, emails, and home addresses. While most people take care not to refer to someone by their real name at events, should it happen, do not take that as an indication that you can do the same until you've earned that right with that individual.

Overall, it is important to pay attention to your surroundings, how people are behaving, and how they (re)act around you specifically. These can be great signals for you to adjust or maintain behavior that you've developed over the years. Remember to allow yourself to be open and accepting, not just in your body language but also in your willingness to adjust your behaviors to better fit in with the social dynamic in which you now find yourself.

Important Note: Some people within the Autism spectrum, such as those with Asperger Syndrome, will have limited or no ability (or otherwise find it extremely difficult) to detect social cues and interpret body language. Additionally, social anxiety is on the rise so this could account for someone seeming jittery or "shifty" even as they are trying to maintain calm and control. Keep this in mind if someone you're speaking with seems to be unaware of any and all body signals that you give off.

Chapter 20

Disorders, Disabilities, and Triggers

O ver the years we all tend to acquire certain aches and pains. Some of us have permanent disabilities. Others have mental or emotional trauma or disorders. Still, others may have past experiences that, if triggered, could result in any number of manifestations. It's time to take a close look at yourself and determine what, if any, of these issues you have because it will be absolutely vital information to your dominant. It's also important for you to be aware of these things in others so that you can be more understanding and helpful to others who experience any one or a number of these situations.

Disorders

Disorders can range from eating disorders, bipolar, anti-social personality, Asperger Syndrome, depression, panic attacks, and the list goes on. Our society is inundated with people suffering or living with all kinds of disorders whether they require medication, therapy, or just self-awareness about their issues and how to avoid problems. If you have (or suspect you have) any disorder you will have to disclose this to the dominant considering you at some point.

Most dominants are very understanding and will accept you regardless of the disorder, but they will need to know what it is and how you maintain it so that they can engage in a healthy dynamic with you. In knowing that there is a disorder and what it entails or how it manifests then the dominant can understand why certain behaviors arise, can avoid engaging any potential triggers, and even help ensure your maintenance goes unhindered. That is to say, if you require medication every four hours they will need to be aware that scenes, events, or even regular outings may require a brief pause to ensure you receive your medication on time. A dominant who is unaware and has you in a long scene that results in missing your scheduled medications could spell disaster.

Also, a dominant may opt not to get involved with you based upon your disorder. This may be due to not having accurate information on their part and misunderstanding what the disorder entails, or it could mean they are not interested in that level of control, care, or maintenance. Some dominants may have come from a background of disorders in their family or past relationships and have developed a wall against engaging with future partners as a result. For whatever reason, some will decline to accept a submissive if they deem the disorder too much to handle or too complicated to navigate through within the relationship. It is better to deal with these issues early-on than to have spent a good deal of time and effort getting to know one another and have it end further down the road.

When disclosing the disorder you should try to provide some general information, but focus on how it applies specifically to you. As with anything else, each person has their own reaction and responses to life and stimuli and a disorder is no different. Is your disorder only a mild case that is easily managed, is it one that might not even surface often, or do you require daily medications and missing a dose could cause a significant issue? If you are on medication for your disorder then this is also very important for the potential dominant to know since many medications need to be taken at certain times, in specific intervals, with/without meals, and can be an issue if alcohol is involved. Not to mention, you will want to disclose that you're taking prescribed medications so that the dominant doesn't think you're doing drugs.

Another important aspect to include in your disclosure is how you react and respond. Are there times when you may require medical attention or even hospitalization? A dominant will need to be aware of this, be able to provide important medical information to EMS or hospital staff, be able to tell them about your condition, and provide a list of your medications.

Some people feel that just by having a disorder they will be shunned from consideration by a dominant or even the community at large and, as a result, will try to hide or withhold that information. Not only is this deceitful but it is dangerous. While you don't need to shout it from the rooftops, you do need to disclose information like this to a dominant with whom you've been speaking or have recently met in person. Besides, if they aren't interested in pursuing a relationship with you based solely on your disclosure then you know straightaway they weren't the right person right from the start. Don't let desperation for finding *a* dominant cloud your judgment in finding the ***right*** dominant.

Disabilities (Physical)

A disability, by its definition, is something that limits your actions or senses. For the purposes of this section, I'll be discussing physical limitations or disabilities. As mentioned, we naturally develop aches and pains through the years and those could be limiting factors. There are congenital (from birth) disabilities and those acquired through accidents or circumstances. Certain medical conditions can create or exacerbate other health concerns like heart problems or joint/muscle pain. Whatever the cause or degree that you experience a limitation, it is also equally important to inform the potential dominant.

Minor Limitations: This includes mild arthritis, general aches and pains, or even something that is chronic but does not overly infringe on your day-to-day life.

This is the one thing people fail to report to a dominant because they often have grown so accustomed to the limitations and have adapted to them within their lives that they almost forget to even mention them. Some might think that since it is a minor or periodic issue it isn't even worth mentioning. However, you are venturing outside your known comfort zones when you get involved in the lifestyle and start engaging in scenes so something that is barely a thought to your daily life, especially something that you've managed to adapt to accommodate, can flare up or worsen by engaging in something BDSM related.

Kneeling is extremely common in the lifestyle. Someone with knee problems, past surgeries, or arthritis who could easily manage normal activities might suddenly find themselves in agony after having knelt for even a short period of time. What was once just a minor ache pushed into the back of your mind could wind up becoming a major pain and ruin the rest of your evening.

Allergies and Asthma: Allergies can be something that you will want to make note of to the dominant and are typically a minor limitation unless you have severe reactions. Allergies can be to any number of things from food, additives, certain scents, to seasonal allergies to bee stings. If you have any allergy, especially one that could result in a severe reaction such as anaphylaxis, it is imperative that you inform the dominant and tell them where you keep your EpiPen or other medication if you have any.

Asthma can range greatly from very mild to sports/exercise-induced to extremely intense and life-threatening. The "attack" can also vary just as widely from just needing a moment to catch your breath to needing an inhaler to even requiring oxygen or emergency response. Once again, do not base your current reactions entirely on your vanilla experiences. An intense scene could make someone who is normally just mildly asthmatic (such as just needing a moment to catch your breath) into someone who will require an inhaler as your breathing can change significantly during a scene. This is especially something to consider if there will be bondage or specific positions involved as being spread out or in certain positions that can make it a little harder to breathe.

Past Surgeries: This is important to disclose even if the surgery has seemingly fixed the problem. If you had surgery on your knees, shoulder, wrists, or even your heart, all these areas (and others) will be put under a unique kind of strain when in a scene particularly ones with any kind of bondage. Cuffs, suspension, prolonged kneeling or standing, specific positions, and even physical exertion will put stress and strain on your body that you haven't experienced before and "fixed" problems could suddenly spark to life once again. Tell your dominant about your surgical history as it never hurts to err on the side of caution.

Prolonged Stances or Overheating: If you had heat exhaustion/stroke in the past you are more prone to experience it again. Sometimes prolonged positions (standing and kneeling) can cause you to overheat even if the weather is fairly mild or the event is indoors. The excess body heat from a crowd at an indoor event could make a warm room suddenly feel uncomfortable or even make the air feel stifling. While you may not be doing a lot of movement that would generate an increase in body temperature, the longer you hold a specific position the more the body must exert itself to maintain it and that energy creates body heat. You may not realize it initially, but the external temperature can rise and when combined with a scene or other exertion you could easily overheat yourself. If you're engaging in activities or scenes in an outdoor space in warmer weather overheating becomes an obvious risk.

Additionally, if you have a circulation problem that could be triggered by maintaining a prolonged position this is equally vital to mention. Blood flow problems could have numerous triggers such as keeping your arms above your head for too long, being bound in certain positions or too tightly, or simply by standing for too long. Any of these could result in the possibility of passing out. Along with the blood flow concern, absolutely make sure you mention to a dominant if you're on blood thinners or otherwise have blood clotting issues. In addition to potential issues as just mentioned, there is always a chance that the strike of a toy/tool could cause a cut even if that's never the intention. Knowing that you're on blood thinners means the dominant can be prepared ahead of time for this possibility.

Permanent Disabilities

These types of disabilities might require the use of wheelchairs, crutches, or canes. They could also include limbs or body parts that have been damaged or even amputated. It is especially important to inform a dominant of this well in advance. If you are wheelchair bound and the dominant lives on an upper floor apartment with no elevators, accommodations will have to be made or it may not be the best match for you in general. If the dominant is looking primarily for a service-oriented submissive with more domestic chores than play/scenes this may also be a problem. This doesn't mean that you would automatically be unable to be submissive to a dominant. Arrangements can be made such as the dominant being willing to come to you or specifically attending events together which are known to be handicap accessible. Adjustments will need to be made so it does need to be addressed early in the relationship. Do be aware, however, that a dominant might opt not to accept you as a submissive based on such limitations for any number of reasons so don't get disheartened, just know that there are others out there who won't have an issue or can be more accommodating.

Triggers

A trigger can be a frightening and complicated situation because you may not be aware of what it is and will subconsciously respond without realizing exactly what caused the reaction. You might feel that the odds of being triggered are small enough or that your response is mild enough to not think about it or that you have adapted and therein don't need to mention this do a potential dominant. Even if you feel your scenes won't involve anything that could be a trigger, the dominant needs to know because it could happen by sheer happenstance.

FOR EXAMPLE:

If someone had a trauma that involved fire and is in the middle of a flogging scene but someone is setting up nearby to do a fire play scene, it might cause a trigger and the traumatized submissive may have a mild to even extreme reaction.

Multiple scenes going on in a play space is fairly common and as long as the event allows for things like fire-play there would be no way for the dominant to realize that such a scene could be a major trigger for you unless it is discussed in advance. That is why it is so important for you to dig deep and address anything at all that could be considered a trigger.

Triggers are often the result of a past traumatic event, but when something in the present hits a little too close to home it could cause a wide range of reactions. Some get defensive, others get aggressive, while others get extremely emotional. Whatever type or degree of reaction you have the dominant needs to be informed. While you don't necessarily have to delve into the psychological background or the details of the triggering event right off the bat, you should at least be able to say something like, "I don't mind wrist cuffs but I can't be bound so I'll hold on to the cross because being bound makes me panic."

Additionally, you may have a triggered response without necessarily realizing it and it could be in response to something fairly mundane. If you've ever had past trauma of being abused you might find that you flinch if someone moves too quickly near your face. It could be that the idea of having a hand on your throat or outright choking is sexy but when you actually experience it for the first time it could cause a significant trigger. Without knowing this is a possibility the dominant could misread your response as "play fighting," especially if you're triggered enough to not be able to use a safe word. A dominant who's been informed of such past trauma and possible triggers would be more apt to go slowly such as starting with just a hand on your throat, then some gentle squeezing, and then perhaps harder squeezing and they'd likely check in with you every few moments to make sure you're present and enjoying the sensations.

Panic Attacks: Panic attacks are similar to triggers since they are often the result of a specific incident or a type of situation. A panic attack can occur without warning and sometimes the cause won't be overt or realized until the situation already passed. Panic attacks can be mild, such as mild hyperventilation that can be easily controlled by stepping outside for some fresh air, to a full-blown event that might require emergency services. Often a person who experiences panic attacks will know that they happen, even if they don't always know why, and will have medication on them or at least know how to help alleviate the attack. If you experience panic attacks it is your responsibility to inform the dominant and tell them where the medication is (including any special instructions on administering it) or how to otherwise assist you through the attack. If you're at an event as a single person or with a friend it wouldn't hurt to advise the organizers or friend where the medication is, especially if large gatherings may be potential triggers.

Once more, I must emphasize that as someone new to the lifestyle you need to plan for and expect the unexpected. Something you see or experience could seem fine, reasonable, and even manageable in theory but when you actually go through it your reactions can be quite the opposite. While a good dominant will try to gauge the reactions of a submissive during scenes they are not mind readers so the submissive needs to provide as much information beforehand as possible.

For someone looking to develop a more long-term or frequent relationship with a dominant, these are important concerns to discuss. In many cases, they should be divulged earlier rather than later as they could be determining factors for the dominant. Purposefully withholding information such as this could also be seen as lying by omission or that you have an inability to communicate, and communication is a vital aspect of our lifestyle. Some might even go so far as to equate you hiding, misleading, or lying about any of these issues as removing their right to consent as you are now forcing them to engage in a relationship, a dynamic, or a scene without the full knowledge needed to ensure that both parties are safe.

Dominants Are Not Immune

I want to keep emphasizing the point that dominants are flesh and blood humans as well and, as such, could easily have past trauma, physical limitations, or ailments. It's extremely important that a submissive turn this chapter around and get to know if the dominant has any of these issues and, if so, how to help the dominant if necessary.

Would you, as the submissive, eventually be responsible for making sure the dominant takes all their medications (including supplements) every day? Will you be responsible for giving massages because the dominant has a bad back? Can the dominant not perform certain scene-related activities such as flogging because they tore their rotator cuff? Is the dominant in a wheelchair and will need specific kinds of assistance? Does a dominant not want to be touched in a certain way because of past trauma?

There could be just as many possibilities with a dominant so it's just as important to make sure you ask questions along these lines. Remember, however, that while you may be comfortable discussing anything about yourself in this area others may have a hard time, so respect the dominant if they say, "Yes, there are some things that will need attention but we can get into that later on," because they don't necessarily want to give away information until they're reasonably sure you aren't going to just disappear or that there's some trust developed.

SECTION FOUR:

MEETING A SPECIFIC DOMINANT

Chapter 21

Phone Contact

Assuming you haven't met yet, such as at public functions, once you've established an online connection and you both feel comfortable, the next step is usually phone contact. This could be texting, voice calls, or a combination of both.

Having a dominant's phone number is not an open invitation to call them all the time. If they haven't given you parameters for calling, simply ask them. You'll score points for showing them that you value their time. The dominant might tell you to only call after a specified time in the evening as they might be working all day and be unable to accept phone calls. They may not even have their phone on them while at work and after a long day they won't appreciate seeing *14 missed calls* from a new submissive panicking because they couldn't reach the dominant while they were at work.

In some cases, when a submissive finally attains this coveted stage in the relationship, they can go into overdrive or even panic mode. Because technology allows us to be in instant and constant contact we have come to expect rapid responses, so if a submissive doesn't hear from the dominant quickly they might feel that the dominant has lost interest or is ghosting them. Paranoia takes over and now the submissive bombards the dominant's phone. This is not reassuring to the dominant and is, at the very least, annoying. A submissive needs to have patience and flooding their phone shows that you have none. Submission can often be a waiting game, whether waiting for the sting of a whip, waiting on your knees, waiting to eat until the dominant does, or just simply waiting for them to respond to your message.

Still be aware of the cues or red flags mentioned in previous chapters. If the dominant states that you can only call on this specific day in this very specific (and very limited) time frame, then you may want to proceed with caution. This is a tactic some online scammers use to allow you to call to "verify" them as a specific person/gender but only during a date and time that the scammer has access to a woman/man who is willing to play their game. However, if you have a broad time frame to call but don't get an answer then chances are the dominant is just busy. The last thing you want is for your potential dominant to get flack at work because **you** did something wrong like calling too often that co-workers or bosses notice.

A Word About "Gender" Verification Calls: While the outrageous number of scammers out there, especially males pretending to be females, does warrant something along these lines, it's important to be aware that some transgender people do not have a voice that you would typically equate with a specific gender. A trans man who hasn't been on HRT may have a voice that sounds like what you equate with women or a trans woman who may have been on HRT for years may have trouble bringing their voice into a higher register. Take gender verification with a grain of salt and if you're speaking to a trans person then be aware that what they sound like might not be what you expected, but it doesn't mean they're any less the gender in which they identify.

Meanwhile, you should try to make yourself as openly available to the dominant's phone calls as possible. Once again, a job might be a hindrance and a good dominant will recognize the need for you to be able to support yourself and won't do anything to infringe on that. However, if your schedule or job setting is more flexible, make yourself as available to them as possible. This might even mean being open to calls at "off" hours such as late at night or very early in the morning.

View this as practice because the entire purpose of seeking a dominant (within the scope of this book) is to serve them and to do so in real life. As such, serving could mean getting up in the middle of the night to get them a drink of water or getting up earlier than the dominant to make sure the coffee is on or breakfast is ready.

Allowing the dominant open access to call you will also help give you some indication of how demanding they might be of your time. If they consistently call and wake you up at ungodly hours and you truly can't stand not getting a full night's sleep, then continuing the relationship further might be counterproductive. Chances are that the dominant's behavior isn't going to change once you take it to an in-house relationship and, in fact, could very well even intensify.

Despite being a dominant, the entire weight of the conversation should not fall to them. Do not leave dead air between you but, at the same time, do not fill silences with, "Um," "Uh," "Ah," and "Hmm," or other highly annoying fillers. This tells a dominant that you were either not paying attention or you don't share enough of an interest in enough things to really be able to contribute to a conversation and could mean you just won't click. If you do not know much about the particular topic the dominant has chosen to discuss you can say: "Sir/Ma'am, this sounds very interesting. I don't know much about it, could you explain it a bit more?" This gives them the sense that you're paying attention, are interested in something they have a passion for, you're receptive to gaining information, and they can freely talk about something they enjoy. If you are paying close attention to the conversation you can take cues from them to expound on something they say or be prepared to answer any questions the dominant asks in an articulate manner.

We all understand that the first time talking to a dominant over the phone (or even in person) can be a little scary and you may get flustered but don't let it get the best of you. Many dominants will understand your nervousness and grant some leeway with stumbling but if you truly have nothing to contribute and make them do all of the talking, there's a great chance they're going to hang up and delete your number.

On the flip side, you might be bursting at the seams to talk to them about everything and anything. Don't monopolize the conversation and whatever you do never, ever talk over the dominant or interrupt them. Granted, a little of this overlap may happen but you, as the submissive, must be the one to cease talking and don't even think of making the dominant be the one to stop. If they say, "Go ahead," you can say **one time**, "Sorry, Sir/Ma'am, what were you about to say?" If they grant you the lead again to continue with your statement do not annoy them by insisting they go first. Simply thank them, make your statement concisely so you can volley the conversation back to the dominant.

Moderating your voice while you're on the phone is also very important. There's no need to holler into the mouthpiece (including and especially when dealing with cell phones) and pierce your dominant's eardrums. Make sure that your environment is not overly loud either such as planes, trains, busy malls, or an open window while driving. All these background noises can and will filter into the call and will either make it difficult to hear you, require you to practically yell into the phone, or just become annoying. When using Bluetooth in the car, be aware of quality issues and keep your windows closed as many Bluetooth setups will pick up the excess noise and drown out your voice. Further, you want to be aware of your environment and the loudness of your voice since you (and the dominant) don't want certain parts of the conversation overheard by random strangers.

Try not to use the speakerphone option since that will automatically create distortion, reduce the voice quality/volume, and could tell the dominant that you're otherwise occupied and are not focusing on them. We can tell when we're on speakerphone because people naturally tend to speak differently and the sound seems further away. If the dominant called you when you were right in the middle of something you can say: "Sir/Ma'am, would you mind if I used speakerphone for a moment while I finish this task?" Although, if it's something that can wait until the call is completed that would be your best option.

Nor is it appropriate to speak so softly that they can't hear you. If the dominant says: "What?" even once take it as an immediate cue to adjust your voice level up a notch. Whispery soft murmurs might be sweet in the bedroom but they actually come across as creepy or sneaky over the phone when speaking to someone for the first time. It says that you're either on the other end of the phone hoping to talk about something good and juicy enough to masturbate to or you're sneaking around trying not to let your significant other who you never mentioned overhear you. Of course, if you have a medical condition that limits your voice range, that's understandable and should have been broached well before you get to the telephone stage. And yes, some enjoy submissives speaking in a meek voice or generally being soft-spoken but that's not always the case and, even if the dominant likes such a manner of speaking, you're not doing it right if they can't hear you and need to keep asking you to repeat what you said. You can speak clearly and with enough volume and still speak softly.

Sneaking around on a significant other is a major no-no and many dominants will absolutely not tolerate such behavior and therein will not get involved with anyone who is willing to sneak, lie, or cheat on their significant other. If you're willing to be deceitful to someone you're sharing your life with on an intimate basis, then how can the dominant trust that you won't be just as sneaky or untrustworthy with them? Moreover, when dealing with BDSM elements, there needs to be a level of trust that exceeds what is usually there in vanilla relationships, and a dominant who is dealing with a sneaky submissive could be putting themselves at great risk.

There are many who engage in open or poly relationships and, in some cases, develop "families" and will intermingle for play or sex within them. If this is the arrangement you have with your significant other and all parties are informed and okay with the new development, that is one thing, but to secretly develop a relationship with a dominant while your significant other is completely unaware is unacceptable. If you are in a relationship and you truly cannot live a vanilla life any longer, then you need to have a very serious conversation with your significant other and do so well before you even start speaking to dominants online.

Everyone has the ability to text these days and while it's not a phone call, it still requires time and effort on the dominant's part to read and respond. Do not abuse this form of contact. There's a great chance that they will have you send a text versus calling and will use calling more for verification or if something needs to be addressed in great detail or with immediacy while the bulk of the conversations will be through text.

Even though you can now text the dominant, whenever you do try to show some personal restraint and don't text too early or too late. If they don't respond to your message right away, even if you see that they read it, they might have just checked the message but don't have the time to respond immediately. That doesn't mean you should bombard them with additional messages and never go the route of: "Are you mad/did I do something wrong?" after the first couple of unanswered texts. This type of text practically demands an answer and by this point you've likely gotten the dominant pretty annoyed with you, so while they might not have been mad at you before, they probably are now.

Feel free to send your morning greeting and wishes for having a wonderful day. If they've instructed you to send a message (of any kind) to them at specific intervals, adhere to that schedule. If they don't respond until that afternoon/evening, thank the dominant for their time and hope their day is going well. You can state that you are available should they wish to chat and then leave it at that. You should always put the ball back into their court where the dominant has control of the situation... After all, control is really the name of the game.

Since texting is intended to be rapid-response, we have developed a specific language called SMS language (as previously discussed). Some are certainly more adept at using it than others but it doesn't matter if you're a texting genius, this is not the way in which to communicate with your dominant. Even if they use text-speech you should always make it a point to spell out all of your words. There's some obvious exceptions such as using LOL, OMG, BTW, and similar acronyms but absolutely avoid lazy texting such as u = you, tho = though, dat = that, tryna = trying to and so on.

Punctuation, in this case, can usually be overlooked, but if you can do it, all the better. Check with the dominant to see if they want you to adhere to any specific writing protocol while texting, such as using lower case letters whenever referencing yourself while capitalizing letters referring to the dominant. This is a universally accepted method of showing submission and more often than not you can err on the side of caution here by doing it unless they specifically state otherwise. However, if you find it difficult to text this way due to autocorrect and it's causing you to waste time going back to "fix" the text then let the dominant know and they might allow you to forgo such protocols when in texts.

The dominant, however, can capitalize, lowercase, or text-speak all they want. If they're very busy and throw out a plethora of abbreviations try your best to decipher them and respond. When in doubt, there are plenty of websites available to teach you what they all mean so you don't have to keep bugging (and potentially annoying) the dominant with, "What does that mean?" or "I'm sorry, I don't understand what you said." Not only did they write it the first time but now you're making them repeat themselves by spelling it completely out when a quick search could have saved the day.

At this stage, you have a certain level of investment in each other and some basic protocols may be in place. If you haven't been doing so already and if the dominant hasn't mentioned it yet then you may want to inquire if they would like you to begin addressing them with a specific title or honorific. You will need to understand that since calls can be overheard in public it might not always be appropriate to use titles or speak in explicit terms. If this happens, you should inform the dominant early in the phone call that you're in a public setting so they understand why you cannot use certain words or answer things as explicitly as they might and you're not simply breaking protocol. Alternatively, texting allows for significantly more privacy but also ask if it is okay for you to use titles or explicit language during those exchanges. Just remember the warning about notifications as mentioned in Chapter 13.

Remember, while you are seeking a dynamic that is rewarding to you and respects your desires just as much as it's about the dominant's desires remember that being submissive and service is tilted toward the dominant, their day, their time, and their being able to do things that you cannot. Such is the life of a submissive and by accepting these tiny things here and there you'll better prepare yourself for the larger acts of service and submission down the road.

Chapter 22

First Meeting

A little word on first meeting safety to help ensure you are both relaxed and can enjoy your time together.

Safety Call: Set up a Safety Call ahead of time with a friend you trust to come and get you or send help if ever needed. You don't have to explain to them that you're meeting a kinky person, you can just say that you're meeting a person you've been talking with online (not at all strange these days) and you just want to make sure you have some safety back-up. This is advised for anyone, regardless of gender or whether they're dominant or submissive. In fact, it's advised to have something like this set up any time you meet anyone from online even if it's a completely vanilla situation. Unfortunately, the world is just too dangerous and getting worse to not take a simple step like this anymore.

Pre-arrange a time that you will call your friend to let them know that everything is okay. It is best that this is a call rather than a text so your friend can know it is actually you on the other end and can even tell by your voice if you're having a good time or there's something "not right" in your tone. Sometimes people will establish a word or phrase as a code that there's a problem but you feel it's not safe to say as much. It should be something not so unusual that saying it will alert whoever you're with but also something not so common that you could say it by accident.

FOR EXAMPLE:

If you absolutely hate banana cream pie you could say: "We're having dessert. I absolutely love the banana cream pie they have here." This is a signal to your friend that things are not quite right and that they should come to get you.

If you miss the predetermined time to call then your friend should try calling you. If you miss two call-backs then your friend knows to come and get you and/or call the police. Obviously, make sure that your friend has the address, date, and time of the meeting. They should have, at least, the dominant's name and phone number. You can inform your dominant ahead of time that you are setting up this arrangement and will need a few moments to make the call, otherwise using the phone in front of them is rude (which we'll discuss in a moment). Alternatively, you can excuse yourself to the bathroom to make the call if you don't want to disclose that you have this setup. For female dominants, don't be surprised if she has made safety call arrangements for herself. If you do disclose to the dominant that you're setting up a safety call and they are offended by your attempts at safety this is a red flag, as any good dominant will understand the world can be a dangerous place and a little precaution does no harm.

Location: More often than not the dominant will likely pick the location, date, and time of your first meeting. First-meet locations should always be somewhere public such as a coffee shop or restaurant. While strolling around the mall or going to a movie are both public locations they aren't advised for a first-time meeting, and things like movies aren't helpful because it doesn't give you an opportunity to actually talk and get to know each other.

Even if you're unfamiliar with the location that the dominant provided there should be no excuse for being late. Between all of the apps that you can use for GPS directions these days, especially now that they're smart enough to indicate traffic issues and offer rerouting options plus telling you how long it will take and what your arrival time will be, there's no reason to be late. To be extra sure that you aren't late you can go to Google Maps and put in the address the day before your meeting to see what the average drive time is, but it also has an option to change the date/time of when you want to arrive/depart by to get estimated future travel times. If you check Google Maps the night before and it says it will take you fifteen minutes to reach the destination then make sure you give yourself at least thirty minutes for travel time to ensure you're not late.

Remember, an ability to think ahead, troubleshoot, and be prepared is highly sought after traits in a submissive and you will surely gain great ground if you illustrate these capabilities.

At no time should the dominant ever have to be waiting for you. Once you arrive, put your name in at the host(ess) stand to request a table so it will be available when the dominant arrives and they won't be kept standing. If they opt to sit at the bar you can then tell the host(ess) that you're sorry for the mix-up but you won't be needing the table. Either way, you were prepared and didn't keep the dominant standing or waiting needlessly. After you put your name in at the stand you may want to scope out two seats at the bar in case the dominant arrives and there's still a wait. At least that way the dominant still has a place to sit while you wait. If the dominant has mentioned that they are a recovering addict then do not take a seat at the bar nor offer the bar as an option unless the dominant tells you otherwise. You should text the dominant and let them know where you are sitting/waiting, especially if you've already been shown to your table. Even though you let them know where you were seated you should keep a close watch on the door as you do not want to have the dominant standing around looking for you.

With the exception of your safety call, once the dominant arrives your phone should be silenced and put away. You are there to give them your undivided attention and learn about each other in the hopes of developing a spark. Unless you have a loved one in the hospital or children at home and you truly need to at least see who is calling/texting, there should be no reason you cannot go without your phone for the duration of the meeting. If something like one of those situations is happening at the moment and you do need to keep the phone out just to make sure there's no emergency, make sure you explain this to the dominant immediately so they understand and don't just think you're incredibly rude. The dominant should also inform you if they might need to take an emergency call at a moment's notice, otherwise the dominant should also show you the basic respect of not using their phone during your conversation. If they say: "Sorry, I really need to take this it's about the kids/sick grandmother/whatever," graciously accept that they have a lot on their plate. However, if they do it several times then you might want to re-evaluate things unless behavior like this doesn't bother you.

That kind of behavior says they care more about their phone than your evening or potential future connection unless it's something you don't really see as being a big deal. Using one's phone at the table is a raging epidemic and has become a social norm, but despite it being ubiquitous do not fall into this practice when you're meeting a dominant for the first time.

Remember those tips about cues and body language? This is a good time to put them to use. If the dominant keeps checking their watch or glancing at their phone on the table, it may indicate that they're bored, disinterested, or that they have something else going on and aren't giving you their full attention. If you see this behavior you may want to make an extra effort to give the dominant time to speak by asking questions or discussing something about which you know the dominant is passionate. Sometimes a direct approach can be just as good as long as it doesn't come off as rude. Saying: "You are obviously distracted so let's call it a night," can be really obnoxious whereas something like: "I really enjoyed meeting you, I don't want to take up too much of your time if you need to get going…" The latter gives the dominant a gracious way out or it calls attention to the fact that they're being less than engaging but either way puts the ball into their court without sounding rude.

Some relationships are built solely around the D/s concept that the submissive (or slave) is to be considered "less than," humiliated, and/or abused. If this is your arrangement and the dominant ignoring you to some capacity is part of that dynamic then enjoy it for what it's worth. Just be aware though, that on a first meeting you really shouldn't be sitting there being ignored since the whole point is to make sure you click well with the other person so leave things like this for future meetings whenever possible.

Speaking of groveling and other submissive-like behavior, this should be kept to a minimum on your first meeting. As mentioned, these meetings are (or should be) in public and thus vanilla spaces so your behavior should reflect that. If you both feel comfortable engaging in a scene or play after the meeting if things go well then having some things with you in the car that you can change into might be an option but it's strongly advised that, no matter how amazing the first meeting goes, you do not engage in play that day and let the relationship have some time to develop. One thing to consider is to have your first meeting at an event or munch where you can be a bit freer to engage in certain submissive behaviors. If you're at a munch this is still a public/vanilla space so adjust your behavior accordingly.

Unless the dominant specifically tells you not to, you can and should offer some level of submission during this meeting in subtle ways. This would include addressing them in a manner of respect such as using Miss/Ma'am/Sir even if they normally prefer Mistress/Master. No one would consider Miss/Ma'am/Sir as out of place as it could easily be assumed to be a business meeting. Another thing that can be done that could be service-oriented without calling any attention to either of you would be to exercise your attention-based skills by paying close attention to what and how they order their food. If you happen to notice if anything is wrong or missing when the plate comes out, this is when you can offer to flag down the wait-staff to request the missing item or to fix whatever was wrong. Paying attention while the dominant orders will also help you to learn not just what they like but specifically how they like it prepared. If you're in a bar then you should be the one to go up to the bar to get the drinks, even if you're splitting the tab. Standing at the bar and waiting to be acknowledged and then waiting to be served, especially in a crowded setting, can be a real pain so this task should fall to the submissive.

One great thing to do that doesn't draw any attention to your dynamic from outsiders is waiting for the dominant to take the first bite before you start to eat. It's actually always good manners to never start to eat before all plates are served but making sure that you don't take a bite until the dominant begins to eat is a lovely and subtle thing. If wait-staff come and ask if everything is okay or if anything else is needed do not answer that everything is fine/nothing is needed but, instead, defer to the dominant and let them make such a statement. Of course, if you do need something then be sure to speak up.

While it might not happen on the first meeting, although it's entirely possible, dominants may have some protocol for ordering food. Some prefer to know what the submissive wants to eat and then they will place the order for them while others will tell the submissive what they want and then expect the submissive to place the order for the dominant. It's typically more common for the dominant to place the order but just be aware that it could go the other way. On future meetings and as you get to know one another more thoroughly, it might get to the point where you don't have to tell the dominant what you'd like to order as they will have learned (or vice versa) and there might even be times when the dominant will order something the submissive might not normally want or even like but will expect them to eat.

Avoid that awkward moment when the bill comes and have this discussed and agreed upon when you are first making the meeting arrangements. In fact, you should check to see if the place has a menu online (most do but some don't) and get a feel for the general cost of the meals and if it seems this is outside your budget range then be honest and let the dominant know that this is a bit much for you; would they consider "this" or "that" alternative and actually give them names of alternatives that are similar to the initial place. That is, if the dominant picked a high-priced Italian restaurant don't pick a cheaper priced Chinese restaurant, stick with something Italian since that's what they picked initially.

Do not wait until the bill is suddenly placed in front of you to find out that it's out of your budget or that you were expecting to split the check. Unless you already intend to pay for the bill entirely then you need to have a discussion beforehand, while you're making the arrangements, about splitting the bill or other arrangements. If money is tight or if you're hoping to split the check for any other reason, this is perfectly acceptable, just be sure to let the dominant know that you'd like to have separate tabs to avoid any awkwardness at the time you're discussing the meeting details. Never ever just expect the dominant to pay the bill.

If you've made arrangements in advance to split the tab and the dominant offers to pay the entire bill then be gracious and offer to leave the tip. Since you're not paying for your half of the bill make sure that you don't low-ball the tip. Tipping 'norms' can vary depending on the state or type of venue and for international readers – tipping can be a big no-no but there are some general guidelines: 10% typically means you weren't entirely pleased with the meal, 15% is around the average, 20% is good service, while over 20% means you were very pleased. If the dominant is paying the tab do not tip anything under 20% and, as a general rule of thumb for life, you should consider always tipping 20% or more as this is often the way wait-staff make a living.

Even if you're meeting in a bar setting you should be prepared to buy at least a round or two of drinks. There are usually two options when hanging out at a bar and that is to pay for your drinks each time you order them or to give your card to the bartender to open a tab. You can put your card on file even if you plan to split the bill but, again, make sure you both know that this is the arrangement ahead of time and not when it comes times to settle the tab. Remember to tip in this setting as well. There are a few options: give the bartender a nice tip right off the bat to encourage more attentive service, leave a couple of dollars every (or every other) drink order, or if you're running a tab then add the tip to the overall bill at the end. If you're sitting directly at the bar and the bartender is the one serving you then the tip goes entirely to them. However, if you're in a bar environment where you still have wait-staff bringing you drinks to a table then remember the tip is split between them so try to be a little more generous. Tipping well is not just something you should do because it's the right thing to do but it's something that may get you a few bonus points in the eyes of the dominant.

Here are a few things to consider if you're in a bar location or if drinking alcohol in general. First, if you know the dominant has a history of addiction do not order alcohol when you're out with them regardless of the location. Second, if you are drinking with your dominant do not overindulge as you could easily say or do something that can embarrass one or both of you. Third, keep in mind that while it might not be a big deal to have some drinks during the first – or even the next few – meetings, some dominants do not allow their submissives to drink alcohol or only allow it under very specific circumstances.

There are some really awesome ways to make splitting the tab easy these days, especially since fewer people actually carry cash on them anymore. There are a few options including ones that your bank may have such as Chase QuickPay (although this is still run through the app Zelle) or others like Apple Pay. Zelle, Payoneer, and Cash App are all options while PayPal and Venmo (which is owned by PayPal) are the biggest ones at present. There is, of course, the Square, a credit card reader that you've likely seen at various businesses. It's a free device to get, but might be a little awkward walking around with it and swiping people's credit cards to get their half of the tab paid back to you. The easiest option is Venmo and can easily be used to help split the tab or anything else that requires sending money to someone else as we continue to transition away from physically carrying cash.

Another thing to consider about the setting of the place, especially if it's a location with which you're unfamiliar, is the dress code. Look up the location online and you will likely find a website and some sites will have at least a couple of images of the facility to give you an idea of the type of place and therein the type of attire you should wear. If you're still unsure or if the place doesn't have pictures (or website as not all restaurants have one still) give them a call to inquire about the typical attire. If it's fairly casual you don't want to show up in a suit or cocktail dress while the dominant is in jeans. Alternatively, you don't want to show up in jeans only to find out you needed to be in a dress or a suit/tie. Even if the location is casual like at a diner, don't show up in a t-shirt. A blouse, polo shirt, or even a solid color shirt is fine, just don't wear something with graphics.

Gifts are generally not required although they can sometimes be appreciated, and while this seems to be done more often with a male submissive meeting a female dominant it can be practiced regardless of anyone's gender or pairing. Be wary of chocolates or sweets in general unless it's something you know the dominant absolutely loves or that they have a sweet tooth. Flowers are a nice benign date gift and while some guys appreciate and enjoy flowers this may tend to be more common when giving them to a woman. If you know their favorite variety you will gain extra bonus points by ensuring at least a few of them are in the bouquet, which shouldn't be that large. Jewelry and other more personal items should be reserved for future dates but do pay attention to things they say, including anything they mention having a real passion for, as it might make an excellent gift if it's simple enough or not too over-the-top. Not only is a gift in general typically appreciated but when it's something the dominant mentioned, even in passing, it shows you are extremely attentive to details and, more specifically, to the dominant's wants and desires.

Also, pay attention to them on your first meeting. How does the dominant dress? What jewelry, if any, do they wear? Is the dominant ostentatious or understated? As you continue with meetings you might be able to learn if they seem to favor one fabric or style of jewelry over another. This will help clue you in to basic details about the dominant so if you get to an in-house situation and they ever ask you to get an article of clothing of such-and-such material/style or even if they ask you to pick something up from the store for them you are already beginning to form the foundation of knowledge about the dominant and their preferences.

When you part ways at the end of the meeting you should always thank them for meeting you and tell them that you had a lovely time. If things went well and you truly would like to continue exploring the relationship tell them as much, but don't spew from the mouth or profess your undying dedication and submission to them right then and there. Don't put pressure on the dominant as you're getting up from the table to set up another date but, instead, allow them time to process how the date went and you can always contact them about another meeting the next day. If the dominant wants to set something up right then and you also want another meeting, it's a great sign so definitely take the opportunity, but let them be the one to broach meeting again at that very moment. When you contact the dominant the next day you can reiterate that you had a wonderful time and would love to see them again. There's a chance you could receive: "I enjoyed the meeting too but I don't think it'll work," or the response you're hoping for: "I had a great time too, Sunday looks good for me."

If you get the "thanks but no thanks" kind of response don't keep harping on it, don't try to beg and plead or try to convince them otherwise. First, if a dominant is doing it on purpose to elicit a begging/pleading response this is incredibly manipulative and unless that's the specific type of arrangement you've already expressed being interested in this is questionable behavior for a dominant. If they are purposefully trying to manipulate you in this manner this is typically someone to avoid as things could really get bad or even dangerous down the road. Second, if they aren't interested then being a whiney pain about it will do nothing but reinforce their decision to not proceed. If this should happen then tell the dominant you appreciate the time they've spent with you and would hope that you can, at least, remain friends. This is especially good if you both are active in the local scene and might wind up at the same events on occasion. You could attempt to ask for feedback on why they are no longer interested but this could be a touchy subject. Even if you're genuinely curious and want to know if there are ways to improve, people typically have a hard time hearing anything negative about themselves and the dominant may just not be interested in getting into details. It could also irk the dominant enough to just ignore you, or it could be something as simple as just not having a spark. Be careful how you phrase such a request though, if you do venture into this territory. Try something along the lines of: "I appreciate you letting me know. I am always looking for ways to improve myself so if you have any feedback it would be greatly appreciated."

Should it happen that **you** weren't pleased with how the meeting went for whatever reason, don't simply disappear or "ghost" the dominant. Be polite and still say that you appreciated meeting them as you're leaving the meeting. Let things settle for a little bit and if you feel there really is no point in proceeding further then contact the dominant to inform them that you had a great time but there just didn't seem to be a match and you'd love to continue a friendship. Again, do not just ghost or disappear – be an adult and use your words whether it's a phone call, email, or text.

If all goes well and you both seem interested in continuing then, no matter how busy your life gets the following day, make sure you touch base with the dominant even if it is just a quick text message good morning or midday asking how their day is going. Not hearing from a would-be submissive for several days after a meeting could easily lead a dominant to believe that you're unreliable or simply not interested. At that point, a dominant will not be interested in hearing any excuses beyond that you were hospitalized or unconscious. Most of us have heard, "Sorry for the delay but things got crazy at work," and any other number of excuses. We don't buy it – especially not these days with the absolute ease in which we can communicate through email and texting. It takes only a few seconds to send a text that says, "I had a great time last night. Things are a bit crazy at work here but I'd love to touch base with you in a day or so." You don't have to go into the explicit details about the cause of your delay as long as you make that contact and they can understand the meeting went well and that you're still interested.

Believe it or not, dominants get nervous on first meetings too. Regardless of how cool or nonplussed they might appear during your date chances are they're still at least a little nervous. Dominants do have feelings, they can be hurt, and they can be just as anxious to find out how it went by your level of interest. Simply disappearing isn't just rude it can be hurtful, so if when it's layered with false or false-sounding excuses it just makes matters worse. If you wouldn't want to be strung along waiting to hear from your date the day after, then absolutely don't do it to someone else. Also, you might want to consider that something you found off-putting might have just been the dominant being nervous so a second date might be a good idea. At the very least, let the dominant know about whatever the thing was that bothered you and perhaps they could clear up any misunderstandings.

Chapter 23

Important Matters to Discuss

*I*t's easy to forget what you wanted to talk about or to get so caught up in chatting that some needful things go unaddressed.

Throughout this book, I have mentioned several things that should be covered during your initial conversations. A whole chapter was dedicated to **Disorders, Disabilities, and Triggers** which is an absolute must area of discussion while other topics were included elsewhere. Now that you're at this more advanced stage in your relationship, let's recap some of those subjects to help ensure a safe and developing relationship.

While these topics should have been touched on or even covered thoroughly online and via emails, there should be a little time during your meeting when medical and scene limitations are discussed face-to-face. As I've hammered on the point in the earlier chapters, it is all-too-easy for someone to misunderstand text on a page or for information to appear overly severe (or not severe enough) with just the written word. Now is the time to really dig into the nitty-gritty of the important topics.

It is extremely important to, not just mention but, ensure both parties are informed, educated, and know how to handle/treat medical and mental limitations. Remembering all the intricate details is difficult to do in a short time, so mentioning these in email and face-to-face meetings can help make sure details are not lost since they are so much more important than anything related to what kind of play you both like or your favorite dishes. Of course, it's easy if neither of you has any ailments whatsoever, but it seems just about everyone has some kind of achy-pain that could flare up during a particular activity. It's best to have this conversation **and** understanding before that can happen and a scene or moment is cut short.

While handicaps or chronic issues are very easy to identify, it's the small bodily complaints that can be tricky but should be given attention as well. As I mentioned in Chapter 20, things you've adapted to or don't think are a big deal could be very important and this needs to be discussed.

While you're exploring the lifestyle you also need to explore yourself. As you're doing your searches for a dominant you can also be doing self-diagnostics to test yourself and your abilities. Instead of sitting on the couch to watch your nightly television, try kneeling in upright and relaxed positions to see how well you can sustain each of those positions. If you find you can't stay in that position for too long then you may want to make a habit of kneeling each night to help develop those skills. If you're out with friends and you have the option to sit or stand, opt to stand and see how long you can do so without starting to fidget or shift foot-to-foot repeatedly.

Don't be afraid to do a little exercise if you aren't already set with a regiment. Even something as simple as walking for 30 minutes each day can do wonders for your body and spend at least a few minutes stretching. There's a wealth of information for beginners on light forms of exercise online that you can search to help get started. Not only is this good for you but many dominants will actually require some form of exercise as a condition or aspect of service.

Aside from the more commonly diagnosed mental ailments and complications, many of us act and react to things in our current life because of experiences in our childhood or throughout our lives. For those of a certain age bracket, many of us were taught and told to bury these events and the feelings associated with them, so you may have even blocked them unknowingly. You might just see it as, "Well, everyone gets smacked around by their father so it's no big deal."

It can be a big deal… Generationally, attitudes have changed. Many from the 1950s to 1970s, even into the early 1980s, were raised with corporal punishment and that was simply the accepted norm. Those from the mid-to-late-80s but especially those from the late 90s and beyond are more likely to come from backgrounds where the parental discipline was a time-out rather than a swat on the butt. It's important to understand that regardless of what was considered the norm, the way we were disciplined as kids could have a far-reaching impact on how we respond to others. If you've never been in a BDSM scene or dynamic before but come from an abusive upbringing this could result in emotions and responses coming up that you never dreamed would happen. As such, this is absolutely something that should be discussed with the dominant.

Speaking of generations, if you are considered to be among one generation while the dominant you're interested in is from another generation this could add an extra layer of complication. If the dominant is older and you hate being referred to or treated as younger or hearing things like: "You're probably too young to know this…" then you will want to talk to the dominant about this and see if this is something they tend to do or possibly just consider dominants closer to your age range. For older dominants who are interested in younger submissives they may make references to things that you just don't comprehend because it just wasn't something you grew up with and that's perfectly fine, but if the dominant asks if you understand don't pretend that you do nor should you blow off anything that the dominant might be trying to share with you. If an older dominant does things a certain way but you know of a better or faster way because you're more in-tune with technology then you can mention the new method as a suggestion but otherwise be understanding if the dominant is not interested in changing how they do something. Alternatively, if you're an older submissive and the dominant is going to expect you to be able to do things on the computer or with your phone then be honest about your capabilities and then find ways to learn how to do those things.

One thing that you should confide to your dominant early on is if there are any allergies or dietary restrictions. If you have a seafood allergy that your dominant doesn't know about and they feed you something from their plate this could be disastrous. There are also many people who are vegan and "mostly" vegan. That is, there are those who hold to every tenant of veganism by not eating or using anything that comes from an animal so that could be a big issue if you're really into wearing leather or considering a lot of our tools and toys are leather-based. There are "mostly" vegan types who don't mind or will tolerate material goods made from animals but will still not eat anything that comes from animals. There are also some who identify as vegan although they will eat some animal-based products but only those they know come from humane farms – such as eating eggs from humane farms. There are vegetarians and pescatarians. There are those who are gluten-free, dairy-free (or generally lactose intolerant), and any other number of dietary lifestyle options. If you're a vegan – in any capacity – and your dominant is an avid meat-eater and expects their submissive to prepare meals this could be a major issue.

As far as allergies and/or fears go it's important to discuss if there are any issues with pets. If you're allergic to cats but your dominant has a few then being around them or in their home could be a miserable experience for you. While many milder cases can be 'put up with' using over-the-counter allergy pills, some may be severe enough that you just can't be near anything cat-related. If you're terrified of dogs and the dominant has any this is something that needs to be known. Are you afraid of all dogs, just certain sizes, or just certain breeds?

Hard & Soft Limits

A limit is a big thing in the lifestyle. Many sites will ask you outright what you consider a limit, dominant profiles might have instructions that you should include your limits in your initial email, or it's a topic that will usually come up within the first few conversations. There is a difference between a hard and a soft limit, there are also things you don't know your opinion on and those will come with exploration. It's important to remember that things you're unsure about don't necessarily go straight to the "limit" category. You need to explain that you don't know what the activity is or how you'd react. A dominant might invite you to a demonstration or have you watch a scene to show you more about this activity. This will allow you a safe avenue to gain more information and then you can decide if it's something you'd be willing to try, something that is a soft limit, or if it truly is a hard limit.

When a dominant asks you what your limits are don't list off a whole bunch of things that you don't like or things that might be considered soft limits. Explain that X, Y, Z are hard limits while A, B, C are soft limits, and maybe L, M, N are things you saw the dominant is interested in but have no experience with so you're not sure just yet.

Soft Limits are forms of play, scenes, handling, or interaction that you don't really enjoy but might be willing to do either to some extent for the sake of pleasing your dominant, something that you want to work toward pushing past so that it's not a limit at all, or something that you will only do with certain people or under specific circumstances. These could include breath-play, knife-play, face-slapping, restrictive bondage, or anything else that isn't something you'd readily engage in but might consider doing under the conditions just previously mentioned. As your relationship with your dominant develops and grows you may establish a level of trust to at least try it once.

Often soft limits are derived from a submissive having an unpleasant experience with the activity in the past or even just having a specific image of the play in their head that's a turn-off. Some dominants enjoy pushing limits (within what's acceptable to the submissive as discussed between them) so if there's something you consider a soft limit because you had a bad experience in the past make sure you explain this to the dominant. With a skilled dominant and established trust something that was previously a soft limit could wind up becoming incredibly enjoyable. It's also entirely possible that no matter how amazing the experience is the activity remains a soft limit and you need to express this to your dominant as well. Dominants have soft limits as well and some dominants might also be willing to push their own personal soft limits for the sake of their submissive.

Hard Limits are things that you absolutely refuse to do no matter how much you want to please your dominant. Many of the hard limits are shared across the board by submissives and dominants alike. These include obvious things like being told to perform an illegal act (like rob a store) and anything to do with underage children. If you do come across anyone into illegal activities such as underage children you need to immediately report the person to the website's administration and call your local police department's non-emergency number to find out how to report this kind of potential criminal activity. Other things that are common hard limits include scat, anything to do with blood, vomit, breath-play, race-play, and so forth. These might seem like they should be universal hard limits but there are those who enjoy these activities so remember YKINMK and don't sound judgmental when talking about things that are hard limits, saying things like, "Anything fucked up like race-play," or "Anything sick like scat…" because it's just obnoxious and rude. People will respect what you do and don't like so you need to respect that people have interests in things that you don't like or may even find stomach-turning.

These are just a few examples and are not meant to be all-inclusive by any means. Hard limits are **not** meant to be pushed by either party under any circumstances. In fact, an attempt to manipulate or push past these hard limits could be a deal breaker and result in an immediate end to the relationship. Once again dominants have hard limits as well and knowing what theirs are could give you a good idea if they are into things you are not into or if they're not into something that you feel you really want when you serve a dominant. If their hard limit is spitting but you love being spit on or if the dominant loves golden showers and that's a hard limit for you there's obviously potential issues here that need to be addressed immediately.

As you can see, communicating early on about these things is important, not just for the sake of seeing if you're a good match, but for safety purposes as well. Obviously, through this, you should be able to see that blathering on endlessly about your likes, dislikes, kinks, and fantasies should take a back burner to some far more important discussions.

A Word About "No Limits"

There are plenty of folks who say they are or want to be a no-limit submissive/slave or to have only the limits that their dominant might have, but in most cases the person hasn't really thought this through. They aren't necessarily considering some of the more extreme things that people could be interested in (and still be legal), they might not consider things like being expected to perform sexually outside of their sexuality (such as a gay man being told to perform sexually with a woman). They might not consider that extreme aspects of the lifestyle exist which can include nullification/castration or breast torture.

There's the *idea* of just doing what you're told because you think it's going to be fun and sexy, and who wouldn't want fun and sexy all the time? However, when you advertise any form of no-limits it's imperative that you really understand that people can come up with some outrageous ideas and some might even include illegal activities. It's best to really think about this before making over-reaching statements.

Chapter 24

Future Meetings

Just because you had a successful first date doesn't mean all your manners should fly out the window. Instead, you should continue to hone and fine tune them. Always look to your dominant for guidance or cues such as whether their facial expression or body language indicates pleasure or displeasure when you do or say something or if they outright tell you where to improve or what they specifically enjoy about you. While we all want to be loved and cherished for the people we are, a submissive must always be on a journey of self-discovery and possess a willingness to change and grow. In fact, any person really should have those goals in mind, but there is an expectation that a submissive should make these personal growths more rapidly, freely, or frequently.

Any additional meetings should also be opportunities for you to begin to increase your level of service to the dominant. Obviously, the more you learn about them the better you can serve and this knowledge comes with time, through observation, and through communication. As a submissive, more importantly, as someone who wants to be their submissive, it is your duty to ask questions that pertain to the dominant and not expect them to do all the work for the "right to own you" or to obtain the "gift of your submission."

Asking about their kinks is a part of the process but should be such a minuscule part that it gets mentioned sporadically unless they want to have a discussion based solely on that topic. Instead, your questions should focus on:

- Their favorite drink(s), favorite color, and favorite food.

- Do they like tea instead of coffee? How do they take their tea/coffee?

- When they get home from a long day at work do they want a bath waiting and, while they soak, for you to prepare dinner? Or do they just want dinner ready or near-ready to be served?

- Do they love to go for walks? If so, do they take them in the morning, on lunch break, or after dinner? Do they enjoy camping? When do they like to go? Any favorite camping or hiking spots?

- Do they have moments when they want to be left alone (i.e. on walks) or do they more often prefer company?

- Before bed, do they have a set expectation like getting a massage or a foot rub? Or, do they prefer to spend some time scrolling around on their phone, playing a game, or reading?

By asking questions like these, and please don't blast them at the dominant all at once, the more you can discover about how good of a submissive you can be to them and what areas you'll need to learn or work on in order to provide the level of service the dominant desires (and deserves). Additionally, some questions might very well give you some insight into their kinks or, at the very least, things they enjoy rather innocuously rather than asking them to list them.

FOR EXAMPLE:

Asking if they like a massage or foot rub before dinner or before bed and finding out they just absolutely love them... and only for the fact that they feel so good and are relaxing could very well play into your personal foot fetish.

The Dominant Is Not There to Serve Your Kink

Again, it's very important that you find a dominant who shares the same interests and kinks as you so that you can create a balanced dynamic. However, just remember service-based relationships such as these means that the submissive is meant to serve the desires of the dominant. Do not go into things with the mentality that you're going to find a dominant who will cater to your personal kinks   because now you're headed into Do-Me territory and that's where you might want to explore visiting a professional dominant who would be more than happy to cater to any kink or fantasy you have… for the right price.

While you might be single and you might lead a pretty busy life, your place should not look like a tornado just touched down. Always keep in the back of your mind that your dominant could come by at any moment and your home should always be ready for them, just as *you* should always be ready for them. While some dominants might have no interest in visiting your home, some just might and if they walk in to see a sink stacked with dirty dishes, take-out cartons piled around the counter, flies buzzing near the trash, and clothes strewn all over, this is not the type of impression you want to make.

How you keep your home should be something you take personal pride in and will be a big indication of how you will keep the dominant's home. The excuse of being too busy usually will not fly because, if you're already too busy to tend to your own home and affairs, then you're telling the dominant that you'll be too busy to take care of them or anything they might need. Even if the dominant never shows an interest or even the inkling of a thought that they want to see your place, always bear in mind it that could happen. In fact, many dominants do not announce their intentions to submissives, so you will rarely get a heads-up or, if you do, it may be with very little advanced notice. So you should always maintain your home as though they could walk through that door at any moment.

Once you have a well-kept home you could invite the dominant over to your place for a home cooked dinner. Don't offer your home too early in the relationship as access to one's home takes a lot of trust from both parties. This is especially the case with a female entering the home of a male. After a couple of meetings and as things seem to be really "clicking," present the invitation to your home but don't push. Let the dominant think about it and if they decline don't get discouraged. It's not like the dominant is breaking up with you, but they are saying they need a little more time before things move to that level. Smile, say thank you and that you completely understand, and then offer to do something in public that they might enjoy.

Even if your future meetings consist mostly of public outings or lifestyle-related events, these are all opportunities to learn and to show the dominant your skills. When out in public a submissive should be alert at all times so that they can do things like opening the door for the dominant, taking/holding packages/bags, and just generally being attentive to the dominant. Every outing is an opportunity to learn more about what the dominant likes, what style or size clothes they might buy, and what they like to eat. Focus on the items and not on how much they spend as their finances, especially in the earlier stages, are absolutely none of your business.

Eventually, you will get to a stage when you will go to their home and they will likely come to yours and this is when you really learn to fine-tune your service skills and learn the minute details of how they like to be served. In a private setting like this, you can engage in protocols and behaviors like kneeling or using honorifics. Be sure to check with the dominant if there are any specific things they would like to see from you at this stage. Perhaps the dominant will want to start integrating things like eye contact restriction, having to ask permission for basic things like using the bathroom, training you on various positions they enjoy, and other more lifestyle-based activities.

As you see more of the dominant it's important to not only take their cues but to ask if there's anything additional they might want you to begin to undertake. Prior to the first meeting, it might not have been *required* for you to address them in a specific manner whereas now this should begin to be integrated into your meetings. They might want you to address them by title when in private or at lifestyle events but might also have a specific way to address them when in public.

Some of these meetings may be exclusively intended to assist the dominant with a project or even chores. It could be that the dominant will invite you to their home and expect you to help fix things, paint a room, bring in the groceries, clean house, or tend to the yard. This may be a form of a trial period where they can begin to gauge your effectiveness, your ability to follow instructions, troubleshoot any problems that might arise, and just get an overall sense of your performance. The dominant might be watching for a variety of things such as:

- Do you need to take several breaks?

- Are you bullish and just plow through the task or do you handle things with care and attention to detail?

- Are you squeamish when it comes to getting dirty or working in an outdoor environment?

- Did you just vacuum the rug and then dust the shelves?

Once the dominant can begin to see how you handle basic tasks, has gained a good sense of how you engage at lifestyle events, and now has the chance to get to know you through regular contact, you can begin to discuss the next phase. Being *officially* accepted as their submissive.

SECTION FIVE:
IN-HOME SERVICE

I want to take just a brief moment here to emphasize the use of the word "home." Not everyone lives in a house. A home can include apartments, townhouses/condos, mansions, trailers, modular units, and so forth. Regardless of the physical structure in which the dominant resides, the place is their home.

Chapter 25

First Time at the Dominant's Home

Fantastic! You've gotten your first invitation to the dominant's home and you should be excited. A move like this shows that the dominant not only likes you but that they want to connect with you further and trusts you enough to let you into their inner sanctum. Don't think it's smooth sailing the moment you step foot into the dominant's house because there's still a chance you can get the boot as things are still a bit tenuous, and while they're willing to explore with you and give things a fair shot, you're likely not wearing their collar at this point.

You should always try to show an interest in how the dominant has arranged their home. Décor is a personal expression and represents a style that the dominant feels a resonance with in some way. This doesn't mean that you should explore every nook and cranny or put your hands on everything but do show an active interest. Find something that you really like and compliment them on their taste. "What a beautiful collection of such-and-such you have, Sir/Ma'am." Collections mean that they have a passion for something enough that they've invested money and time into establishing a collection, so it's usually a safe bet to compliment and is also something to keep in mind should you ever need to get them a gift.

Be prepared for a chaotic household as well. Not every dominant lives in a big place so you might be walking into an apartment that's chock-full and seems disorganized. While your home should be kept with the utmost care the dominant has some leeway here and, in fact, chances are that one of the purposes they will have for a submissive is to help them get organized and run a clean, smooth home.

While I mentioned you should compliment the dominant on their home you do not, under any circumstances, want to mention any disarray. Even if they say something like: "Sorry for the mess," simply say, "Oh, I don't mind, Sir/Ma'am," and leave it at that. Scoffing at the mess, commenting on it, or in any other way drawing attention to the matter should be avoided. However, if you find that the home is beyond messy or cluttered and is outright disgusting then you might want to take this as a warning. The dominant might have a hygiene problem if you are assaulted with foul odors, see insects, extensive staining on surfaces, or other similar signs. This is not the home of a person who is just too busy to pick up the laundry and put it in the basket nor is that even someone who is a little bit of a pack-rat. If the place is filthy versus just disorganized or cluttered, you need to re-evaluate your own position. They might want you to come in and clean the place top to bottom and you might think the dominant is worth it enough to even try to do such a deep clean. But if they refuse to let you throw anything out or the place is in shambles a few days later, this is not a healthy environment or mentality and the hygiene issues could easily extend to their body or toys. There would be no way to tell if they used that whip or flogger on someone else who might have bled on it or, at the very least, sweated on it and the dominant never cleaned it properly.

Do not invite yourself to sit down as you should wait for the dominant to indicate for you to do so or they may instruct you to sit on the floor or kneel. In fact, even if they sit down, you should remain standing in some form of relaxed attention until otherwise instructed. Do not shuffle or fidget as it's both unsightly and could be seen as you "silently" bugging them to let you sit. Some dominants might purposefully make you stand longer the more you fidget. The exception to this is if you have a medical condition that limits your ability to stand and this should have already been discussed (as mentioned earlier).

There's a good chance the dominant might be testing you or it could be that they simply haven't given it a thought. If they do invite you to sit with something as simple as: "Have a seat," then you can ask them to clarify if they mean in a chair or on the floor. Some of these details might have already been discussed, such as if a submissive is ever allowed on the furniture. If they have, then adhere to whatever rules were previously discussed, but sometimes topics and little details such as this don't actually arise until you're in the moment for the first time.

If the dominant asks if you'd like something to drink, whether you want anything or not, you should offer to get one for them, even if you're in their home. You can explain to them that if they just tell you where they keep the glasses you'd love to serve them a drink so that you can better learn (hands-on) how to serve them. At some point, you're going to be expected to know where everything is, what they drink, ice or no ice, etc. Much of the new meeting jitters should be over at this stage and, as you're in a private setting, you can offer as much service as possible. It starts with simple things like fetching a drink. It goes without saying that should the dominant ever come to your home that you should offer them a seat and something to drink without hesitation.

The subject of play (scene) at this point can become touchy, especially if you haven't discussed it up to this point. It's always good to go into any new situation with your dominant with an open mind, particularly when they haven't made any distinct statements one way or the other. Do not show up at your dominant's house with your toy bag, looking for her toy bag, asking where the dungeon is, or expecting play of any kind. Additionally, you should never appear in any clothing (or lack thereof) that could be seen by neighbors and cause hassles. If the dominant instructs you to come to their house nude, dressed in a maid's outfit, or decked-out in leather, then be sure you have an overcoat or baggy sweatpants over it to provide some discretion.

Do not close your mind to the possibility that the dominant might suggest a scene, even a small one such as a spanking, just to see how things feel on that level. Unless they explicitly tell you to come prepared to scene you should enter their home with the impression that you're there to learn about each other and enjoy each other's company and are getting one step closer to earning their collar.

Further, the subject of sex can be equally, if not more, daunting during these first few in-home meetings. Once more, never expect it, but be prepared. Men and women should have a **new** condom on hand – even if you're meeting up with a female dominant as you should also put condoms over sex toys. Do not use one that's been sitting around for a long time as they tend to deteriorate and can be defective. Even this can be a bit of a catch-22 as being prepared is a good thing but by having the condom on hand could imply you harbored expectations of sex. It is always best to err on the side of caution and, in this case, safety. You may have already discussed that this is going to be a non-sexual relationship. It may be a relationship with sexual aspects but no intercourse. Then again, it may be a full-blown and highly sexualized relationship. Come into this with the cues or statements that the dominant has made leading up to this moment and that means paying attention to their cues, not your personal desires.

There is no time frame for when an in-home invitation will come, when play will start, or when sex will happen (if ever). You might find yourselves in a whirlwind romance where you've had several meetings in public smashed inside of two weeks and you're suddenly at their home, naked and bound to the bed by the start of the third week. Alternatively, you may find yourselves being cautious, enjoying the courtship, and keeping your options open where you meet once a week for dinner or drinks, perhaps occasionally meet at a group event, and maybe months later get your first invitation to see their home, have a scene, or be intimate.

I do want to share a word of caution in regard to the whirlwind romance scenario. Given its very nature, it can become very easy to lose sight of safety and this includes allowing yourself time to process all the new experiences. Heavy and intense situations will eventually require a decompression period so that you can process the sudden flood of information and sensations. This is a prime opportunity for a "crash" to occur and it can sometimes get ugly, especially when it comes to emotions. If you're in that whirlwind romance then, by all means, enjoy it but you need to have a little downtime. If the dominant wants to see you five days in a row then you might want to try to split up the days and have a day all to yourself somewhere in the middle for processing time. This is especially recommended following a heavy scene or something that was new or otherwise intense. If that is the case it's important that you still maintain a level of contact with the dominant, but you should take some personal time, even spend a night out with some vanilla friends for a few drinks or just hanging out at home.

It's very easy to become involved in the lifestyle and a new relationship to the exclusion of all else. While this isn't necessarily a bad thing and even vanilla courtships go through this "honeymoon" period where friends usually fall to the wayside for a while, we are dealing with a whole new level of sensations and emotions than a typical vanilla relationship would ever encounter. Do not burnout within the first month of your new relationship. Even if you want to see the dominant every single day you should still try to break it up perhaps by scening some days while others could be spent at the beach just relaxing or a trip to the stores where you can hold their bags or just go for a bite to eat. You have to be responsible for your own mental well-being. While dominants will eventually learn to read your body language and gauge when you're overstimulated or exhausted, they're not mind readers. If a dominant implies or even asks if you're feeling okay it might be a sign that you need a quick time-out. If the dominant is inquiring like this it could be that they're picking up on signals you're not even aware of, and even if you feel fantastic it could be euphoria masking things like exhaustion so be honest and schedule a little "me time" for yourself to help you recharge.

Alternatively, be aware that dominants can experience burnout as well. While you may be charged and ready to go every single day don't get upset if a dominant does some things on their own. Don't forget that they also have friends and family who would like to see them and there are things in their own lives that they have to tend to just like you so don't freak out if they take some private time.

Chapter 26

Serving the Dominant

So your dream has come true and you are now technically in-service to a dominant. Now is the time to get down to the business of actually serving them, exploring your submissiveness, and learning in a real hands-on environment about the lifestyle. Even if you have prior experience, even if you're a regular at groups and events, the reality of actually serving a specific person is truly a horse of a different color.

This chapter is not going to focus on specifics as every dominant is different and they will train you according to how they want to be served. Whether you're an old-hand at serving or a blank slate, you should try to prevent any preconceived notions from getting in the way of what the dominant is teaching you. This absolutely, positively includes anything you've seen or read online, as it is predominantly fantasy and a load of hogwash and this is why I dedicated a chapter on discussing what is/who are dominants.

I do, however, want to touch on some things you can expect from the dominant and some things they might be expecting of you, at least in a general sense.

Communication Is Key!!!

This cannot be emphasized enough! If you go to any group, message board, chat, or speak to any individual all will tell you the secret to success is the ability to communicate openly with their other half regardless of their dynamic. Do not have an idea in your head and ever expect the dominant to just know what you're thinking. Do not do something that you're petrified of thinking you can get through it because it's what they want without talking to the dominant. Do not put yourself into a position where you are trying to push yourself past personal limits (mental or physical) without informing the dominant. Not only can something like this needlessly ruin a moment but it can also ruin the relationship or even create a dangerous situation. You need to be able to discuss any apprehensions or concerns you have, to ask for details about what any activity might involve, and even be able to state that you're actually uncomfortable with something. If you do not relay this information to the dominant they will naturally work on the premise that everything is okay and will continue down the same road. Once again, dominants aren't mind readers.

You can expect to discuss, without reproach, your hard and soft limits and know they will be respected, as I mentioned earlier. Informing the dominant about limitations also means you won't be expected to perform tasks beyond your capabilities nor will you be punished for an inability to do certain chores or tasks. If you cannot lift heavy objects because of a physical limitation then your dominant won't expect you to carry in that huge box from the car.

You can expect the dominant to tell you to do things that you might think should be done in a different way or that you don't even see the purpose of doing in the first place. As you begin your service you might not understand the methodology that the dominant is using but odds are there's a purpose. If you present the dominant, in a very respectful way, with an alternative method of doing a task (especially one you're expected to do regularly) that's more cost and time effective and emphasize that it will allow you more time to be at their beck and call, there's a chance the dominant will appreciate the input and may even allow you to implement your changes. Then again, they may be steadfast in wanting something done in a specific way so you will need to accept it and do it accordingly even if it still doesn't make much sense to you.

Now that you are officially serving the dominant, whether you've earned their collar or are still working toward it, this is the stage in the relationship where your life and mind need to revolve around them. Everything you do, especially if you're living together, needs to be from the mindset of putting the dominant's needs and desires first and foremost. While reality does like to come crashing in and you might not always be able to put them above all else, your goal here is to at least try whenever possible to be aware that in this dynamic and, as such, typically their needs come before yours.

FOR EXAMPLE:

While you were un-owned there was never a second thought about going to get something from the kitchen, whereas now you should either ask for permission to do so or at the very least, ask if you can bring the dominant anything while you're there.

Some dominants will have you living a relaxed lifestyle where you can essentially go about your day as you would before being their submissive, with a few exceptions here and there. Others, however, thrive on strict protocol and rules. If you're at this point you are well and truly aware of how they like to run things and you've accepted those terms. That doesn't mean you won't continue to discover things about the dominant (and yourself) along the way, as the lifestyle and the people in it are truly growing creatures. Something that might have seemed uninteresting before might now become a new interest or even grow into a new passion. Let the lifestyle take you where it wants and enjoy the discovery.

Any relationship, by its very nature, is an ever-changing dynamic. There's an early period where everything is fresh, new, and exciting which most people call the "honeymoon period." There's the settling in period where you've begun to establish routines. There's even the lull where things can become so routine it starts to become boring. This is where communication is vital because that lull can make or break a relationship. Do not enter a D/s type relationship expecting non-stop action and fun. It is just like any other relationship that takes time to cultivate and will go through its highs and lows, but it's important that you work jointly toward the same goals rather than growing in different directions.

Perhaps most importantly you must be aware of the type of dynamic you're entering into with this dominant. Some will want a submissive only and absolutely no expectations of romantic involvement and even, in some cases, no sexual play or release at all while you're together. Others may be looking for their lover, partner, and submissive all rolled into one where the life partner and submissive aspects can be incorporated and woven into your lives to various degrees. Still, others will say they're looking only for one or the other but as time goes by the dynamic changes as you both grow, whether it's closer together or further apart.

By now you should be learning the intricacies of serving your dominant and continually working, learning, and growing to please them. This is not the time to stop learning, stop growing, or become complacent. It is quite the opposite. You should constantly be looking up how-to articles, books, videos, and other helpful resources. Ask your friends to see if they have any specific skill(s) in an area you'd like to learn more about and if they'd be willing to let you pick their brain for a bit. Explore local resources like the library or online for free or low cost courses.

Your dominant might require a daily massage before bed and while you're 'passable' at performing this task, your ultimate goal will always be to improve your ability to please them, so learning how to give a relaxing massage versus an erotic massage is something you can lavish on your dominant as you learn more about the different techniques and they will undoubtedly appreciate the continued willingness to not just "get by" in your service to them, but in your enthusiasm to improve that service. If your dominant is a vegan then exploring various websites to learn more about it and pulling up recipes to try will go a long way toward pleasing them. Not good at cooking? Ask some friends or pick up a course at a local school (or online) to pick up some tips. In fact, there are an overwhelming number of cooking shows and an entire network dedicated to cooking not to mention the number of channels on YouTube or apps. It might also be a good idea to research butlers or even take a part-time job with a cleaning service to learn more about domestic-based services.

Regardless of the "what," you should always be learning. Pick a random topic that you hear in conversation, on the news, or even from a movie and then go look it up to learn a little bit more about the subject just to keep your mind growing. Is your dominant a big fan of art but you can't tell a Monet from a Manet? While this topic can be a very dry or boring subject for many, there are some wonderful biographical films and documentaries about the subject or many artists. When you were in school you were forced to limit your research to only text-based reading material, but we're not in high school anymore, so you can use movies and videos to help you at least obtain some general information about the subject. Do remember, however, that many films will stretch or gloss over the truth for the sake of making the film more interesting so don't take the information from films as hard facts. Still, it might provide you with enough insight for basic conversation or be the spark for you to seek out more accurate details.

You won't have the exact same interests or the exact same passion for shared interests, so find your common ground and build from there. Be willing to explore things that your dominant is interested in and you might find yourself falling in love with some of those same things.

Chapter 27

Congratulations and Resources

<u>Good Luck</u>

Congratulations! I am congratulating you on successfully reading this book and allowing the ideas and suggestions to enter your mind and to be considered. One of the first hurdles we must all overcome whenever we are striving for a goal is to understand the process we need to take in order to get to those end goals. Since you did just that in buying this book and completing it you are showing a genuine interest in following some basic steps to improve the possibility of obtaining your ultimate goal... serving a dominant.

Whether you've read this book all in one sitting or you've used it as a play-by-play guide by reading a section at a time as you complete the suggestions made in each chapter doesn't matter. The thing that does matter is your stick-to-itiveness and willingness to change behaviors, fix a lack of behaviors, and even adjust aspects of your own personality in order to better yourself, especially in the eyes of dominants. As I mentioned earlier, it's important to not lose yourself so don't make changes that you're uncomfortable with just because you think it will help you get a dominant. If you're unhappy with yourself and aren't making changes for yourself and your own betterment, people will sense that and it will be equally off-putting.

In fact, perhaps the largest problem dominants face is rigidity or stagnation. This seems to be a more common issue amongst men since they are often conditioned to believe they must be strong and sometimes they mistakenly believe "strong" to mean unyielding, unemotional, and even cold-hearted. Now that you've finished reading this book and have taken some steps towards change it opens a great many things that you might not have otherwise had the opportunity to experience.

Remember BDSM and all its many shapes, styles, forms, and intensities are based on a **Power Exchange** and not a power struggle. While a little extra push and pull might be fun on occasion and a little "brattiness" can bring some excitement to your lives, there should not be a constant fight just to maintain your established D/s roles. If that is the case and it's not something either/both of you enjoy then you need to have a serious conversation and re-evaluate the relationship.

However, we're going to focus on the good here and as my favorite bard said: "Sap up the wrap-up."

If you've managed to find the dominant who you wish to serve while you've read this book or because of reading this book, I want to also give you special congratulations. Finding a dominant who fulfills your dreams is a difficult task, with or without help, so I hope this book provided you with some genuine guidance in your search and success. Also, I'd like to invite you to share your success story with me so feel free to reach out and let me know about your success story. My contact information is at the end of this book.

Continued Learning Sources

You've already taken the first step by reading this book to increase your knowledge and you're showing initiative that you want to learn so there's no reason to stop now. I've collected a few resources to continue your education, including some places you may not have thought to look or sources to tap.

Search Engines: I've mentioned this tool throughout the book but it really is an invaluable avenue of information. This is a fairly obvious source of information and it's available to everyone. Typing in keywords will offer you a plethora of sources to explore and I've even mentioned a few keywords to consider checking along the way. There are numerous search engines available and everyone tends to have their favorite. If you need variety in search results then consider trying different search engines.

Also, check your search engine settings as they could be preventing all or limiting "adult" content results and since we're dealing with BDSM some helpful sites might get stuck behind that filter.

Video Sources: We are all well aware of major hubs like YouTube but don't forget others like DailyMotion or Vimeo. Almost as comprehensive as a search engine, you can find almost anything you desire to learn through one of these venues. Massage techniques, cooking, and even how to fold clothes are just a click away. There's also a slew of videos pertaining to the lifestyle from basic concepts to advanced discussions.

Library: While it might be rare, some libraries do carry some books on the lifestyle. If your local library does, then, by all means, tap this resource. However, you will probably want to focus on other more benign subject matters when using this resource. Once again, massage books are in plentiful supply. However, personal grooming, computer skills, increasing vocabulary, household matters, cooking, socializing, organization, and countless other helpful topics can be found here. Use this invaluable resource especially since it's free. Many libraries offer classes for free or extremely low cost ranging from computer skills to communication to psychology/counseling or even knitting and other crafts. Go to them! Remember, most libraries are within a network so they can request books and materials from other libraries to be shipped to that location.

D/s Sites: There are some wonderful sources of real information about the lifestyle out there. Stay away from known or suspected pornography sites, even if they claim to have BDSM on them. Search for sites that discuss personal relationships or provide actual information. You would do well to find sites that have journal entries, blogs, or otherwise focus on specific people/couples talking about their personal lives in the BDSM lifestyle and the things they've learned along the way.

Friends: You needn't 'come out' to your friends about your kinky desires, but if you know someone who has a special skill or talent in a particular field ask if they'd be willing to mentor you. This could include any number of things like cooking, woodworking, handyman skills, or even haircutting.

Bookstore: What you cannot find in the library you can almost always locate at the bookstore or online book sources. If the store itself does not have the item you're looking for they can usually order it for you. Some will allow you to enter your request online so you don't have to feel awkward placing an order for a D/s book but don't let that be the only topic you search. Explore the different sections and see if you can find at least one book in each section that you could learn something from and don't shy away from the self-help section.

Subjects to Look For

I mentioned a few already but I want to reiterate some and suggest a few others.

- Technical knowledge is not just helpful it's almost mandatory now. If you're a little on the older side or just generally not that savvy you will definitely want to look into books and videos to help you in this area.

- Cooking is also a major one as many dominants like to be pampered by having meals prepared for them (although some truly love to cook and will not let you do this for them.) Don't forget baking as the smell of fresh baked goods is bound to put everyone in a pleasant mood and always taste yummy.

- Also, once more, massages, as most dominants will truly enjoy luxurious rubs ranging from gentle, to deep muscle, to erotic.

- You should also look into books or videos about butlers, maid service, and, very importantly, etiquette.

- Organization – helping a dominant remain organized and keeping a household running smoothly is very important. This can also be in conjunction with technology skills as there are many useful apps and online calendars that can help maintain organization.

- Increasing one's vocabulary is always a good idea. Check into a Word of the Day, crossword puzzles, word search puzzles, or even like/follow Facebook pages like 'Grammarly' or 'For Reading Addicts.'

- If you find that a dominant you're speaking with is really into a specific subject then read up on it. This could include music, art, history, movies, or anything else under the sun.

Do not limit yourself in your quest for knowledge.

As you can see there are plenty of avenues and topics for you to explore in your quest for knowledge and personal growth. The lifestyle isn't all about how to be beaten, how to present a plate, or in which position to kneel. In fact, it encompasses so much more and the most important thing you need to focus on is making a connection with someone. As I've mentioned numerous times before, dominants are people and they have non-kinky interests and passions. The more you broaden your own mind and horizons the more people with whom you can connect. Besides, the more skilled a submissive is, the more sought-after and valued they are to a dominant.

In the end, whether it's for a dominant or not, learning is never a bad thing and you should go into it knowing it will benefit you in the long run and a better you is always a good thing.

Specific Resources

How to do laundry: Despite what you might have been told, laundry can be done on the cold/cold setting with some material-specific exceptions. Of course, refer to your dominant on how they prefer their settings or if there are any specific garments that require specialized settings. Otherwise, stick with the Cold/Cold setting as it is more eco-friendly.

- https://www.ehow.com/how_46_laundry.html
- https://www.thespruce.com/how-to-do-laundry-2146149

Butlers: This is for actually attending school to be a butler but you might find it worth inquiring for details on butlers of "today" or for additional research material. There are also a lot of videos available on butler services.

- https://www.britishbutlerinstitute.com/butler-school/

Making the bed: This isn't just simply pulling the covers up. While dominants will likely have a specific way they like their bed made, here are some quick helpful tips in general.

- https://www.wikihow.com/Make-a-Bed-Neatly

Setting the table:

- https://emilypost.com/advice/table-setting-guides/
- https://www.realsimple.com/holidays-entertaining/entertaining/how-to-set-a-table

Etiquette: Where better to go for this resource than the woman herself? Emily Post and the next generation(s) have an invaluable Internet resource on how to present oneself in all kinds of situations. You should view this resource thoroughly.

- https://emilypost.com/

Giving a Massage: You should learn about the muscle groups and how to properly apply pressure.

- (*Video*) https://youtu.be/0SLGvlDVkRA
- (*Video*) https://youtu.be/ocioXi-8TY4

Organizational Skills: Not only are these skills important in your everyday life but dominants tend to appreciate these skills in submissives. To help learn great ideas on cleaning, organizing, spotting trouble spots and so forth use this site for guidance

- Unclutter - https://unclutterer.com/archives/

North Carolina Resources

A few of these were mentioned in the events sections but here is a more expanded list:

Female Artists of Domination (FAD):

Contact Method: Fetlife group: https://fetlife.com/groups/2789

Description: FAD is one of the longest running female dominant groups in the area. They host monthly meetings/events and periodically host special events or themed parties. While this is a female dominant group, just about everyone is welcome with some conditions. Be sure to ask the officers for further details. (Membership required)

Rope Practice Raleigh:

Contact Method: Fetlife group: https://fetlife.com/groups/44047

Description: A safe place to mix and mingle while learning about rope and knots. Casual and informative, Rope Practice Raleigh hosts monthly meetings based on classes and free-form rope-play. (No membership required). *See Chapter 13 for more details.

PUSH!:

Contact Method: Follow PeteCock or Secretarygirl on FetLife

Description: Held quarterly in the Durham area, this is a large-scale fetish party. This is a one-night event with play space, demos, music, and lots of fun mingling. (No membership required) *See Chapter 13 for more details.

Other Resources

Gloria Brame

Contact Method: https://www.gloriabrame.com

Twitter: @DrGloriaBrame

Description: As previously mentioned, Dr. Gloria Brame is a leading sexologist and expert witness. She has dedicated much of her life to sex and normalizing sex and sexuality, including BDSM.

National Coalition for Sexual Freedom (NCSF)

Contact Method: https://ncsfreedom.org

Description: This amazing organization has been around for over 20 years with the primary purpose "…to fight for sexual freedom and privacy rights for all adults who engage in safe, sane and consensual behavior." They currently have over 50 partners and their site offers significant resources and should be a place you keep bookmarked for repeated reference.

More Than Two

Contact Method: https://www.morethantwo.com/polyamory.html

Description: This page specifically gives you a quick rundown on what polyamory is and isn't. They also have a book on the subject that you might want to check out which you can get through the site.

Kink Academy

Contact Method: https://www.kinkacademy.com

Description: This site has a mind blowing number of videos – for free, experts in a variety of areas, and a full blog section. However, if you want complete access you will have to join and pay for the access. Check it out and consider a subscription because like I keep saying – it's always a good idea to keep learning.

Find A Munch

Contact Method: http://findamunch.com/

Description: This is NOT just for munches. The site allows you to search by state or even other countries and lists a variety of munches and groups in alphabetical order. Links aren't verified that often so you may run into a few dead links, so if you find a group that sounds interesting be sure to check FetLife for them as you may find current group information there. This is a fantastic place to start though, especially if you think there's never anything happening in your area.

Leather and Roses

Contact Method: http://www.leathernroses.com/

Description: The moment you enter this site you will be greeted with a substantial list of resources including some humor. This is a good place to save for repeated viewing because there's a lot to read through.

New England Leather Alliance (NELA)

Contact Method: https://nelaonline.org/

Description: They are "...dedicated to making a safer world for BDSM practitioners through advocacy, education, and charitable giving." They're also the group behind the HUGE Fetish Fair Fleamarket that I've mentioned earlier. It's held twice a year and you can follow details about that directly at: http://fetishflea.com

Flag Citations

Gay Flag –

Wikipedia: https://en.wikipedia.org/wiki/File:Gay_flag.svg

Bi Flag –

Wikipedia: https://en.wikipedia.org/wiki/File:Bi_flag.svg

Bear Flag –

Wikipedia: https://en.wikipedia.org/wiki/File:Bear_Brotherhood_flag.svg

Lesbian Pride –

Twilight Guard: http://www.thetwilightguard.org/tg_flags.html

Trans Flag –

Wikipedia: https://en.wikipedia.org/wiki/File:Transgender_Pride_flag.svg

Leather Pride –

Wikipedia: https://en.wikipedia.org/wiki/Leather_Pride_flag

BDSM Pride –

Informed Consent: https://fetlife.com/groups/29263

How to Contact Jude Samson

Share Your Stories

Jude invites you to email him with questions, comments, and suggestions for possible inclusion in new editions. He also welcomes any reviews and is always looking for ways to make the book more inclusive, user friendly, and more fun to read. If you have a success story where you feel this book helped you in your D/s relationship (finding/maintaining one) please share, he would love to hear of your happily-ever-after.

For direct email contact:

SirJudeS@gmail.com

or find him on FetLife under username SirJude:

https://fetlife.com/users/8699

www.ingramcontent.com/pod-product-compliance
Lightning Source LLC
Chambersburg PA
CBHW060300100426
42742CB00011B/1824